System requirement

- Window XP or above
- Windows media player 10.0 version or above (software)
- Power DVD player (software)
- Accompanying CD ROM is playable only in Computer and not in CD player.

CD CONTENT

The Technique of Recording an ECG

ECG Made Easy

Third Edition

Atul Luthra
MBBS MD DNB
Diplomate
National Board of Medicine
Physician and Cardiologist
atulluthra@sify.com

JAYPEE BROTHERS
MEDICAL PUBLISHERS (P) LTD
New Delhi

Published by

Jitendar P Vij
Jaypee Brothers Medical Publishers (P) Ltd
B-3 EMCA House, 23/23B Ansari Road, Daryaganj, **New Delhi** 110 002 India
Phones: +91-11-23272143, +91-11-23272703, +91-11-23282021, +91-11-23245672
Rel: +91-11-32558559 Fax: +91-11-23276490 +91-11-23245683
e-mail: jaypee@jaypeebrothers.com, Visit our website: www.jaypeebrothers.com

Branches

- 2/B, Akruti Society, Jodhpur Gam Road Satellite
  Ahmedabad 380 015
  Phones: +91-79-26926233, Rel: +91-79-32988717, Fax: +91-79-26927094
  e-mail: ahmedabad@jaypeebrothers.com
- 202 Batavia Chambers, 8 Kumara Krupa Road, Kumara Park East
  Bengaluru 560 001
  Phones: +91-80-22285971, +91-80-22382956, +91-80-22372664
  Rel: +91-80-32714073 Fax: +91-80-22281761, e-mail: bangalore@jaypeebrothers.com
- 282 IIIrd Floor, Khaleel Shirazi Estate, Fountain Plaza, Pantheon Road
  Chennai 600 008
  Phones: +91-44-28193265, +91-44-28194897, Rel: +91-44-32972089
  Fax: +91-44-28193231, e-mail:chennai@jaypeebrothers.com
- 4-2-1067/1-3, 1st Floor, Balaji Building, Ramkote, Cross Road
  Hyderabad 500 095
  Phones: +91-40-66610020, +91-40-24758498, Rel: +91-40-32940929
  Fax:+91-40-24758499, e-mail: hyderabad@jaypeebrothers.com
- Kuruvi Building, 1st Floor, Plot/Door No. 41/3098, B & B1, St. Vincent Road
  Kochi 682 018 Kerala, Phones: +91-484-4036109, +91-484-2395739
  Fax: +91-484-2395740, e-mail: kochi@jaypeebrothers.com
- 1-A Indian Mirror Street, Wellington Square
  Kolkata 700 013
  Phones: +91-33-22651926, +91-33-22276404, +91-33-22276415, Rel: +91-33-32901926
  Fax: +91-33-22656075 e-mail: kolkata@jaypeebrothers.com
- Lekhraj Market III, B-2, Sector-4, Faizabad Road, Indira Nagar
  Lucknow 226 016
  Phones: +91-522-3040553, +91-522-3040554, e-mail: lucknow@jaypeebrothers.com
- 106 Amit Industrial Estate, 61 Dr SS Rao Road, Near MGM Hospital, Parel
  Mumbai 400 012
  Phones: +91-22-24124863, +91-22-24104532, Rel: +91-22-32926896
  Fax: +91-22-24160828, e-mail: mumbai@jaypeebrothers.com
- "KAMALPUSHPA" 38, Reshimbag, Opp. Mohota Science College, Umred Road
  Nagpur 440 009 Phone: Rel: +91-712-3245220
  Fax: +91-712-2704275 e-mail: nagpur@jaypeebrothers.com

ECG Made Easy

First Edition: 1998
Second Edition: 2004
Third Edition: 2007
Reprint: 2008

ISBN 81-8061-946-x

Typeset at JPBMP typesetting unit
Printed at Ajanta Offset & Packagings Ltd., New Delhi

To

My Father

Mr PP Luthra

Who made me

and

My Mother

Ms Prem Luthra

Whose memories

Still guide me

PREFACE

The imaging techniques of contemporary 'high-tech' cardiology have failed to eclipse the primacy of the 12-lead ECG in the initial evaluation of heart disease.This simple, cost-effective and readily available diagnostic modality continues to intrigue and baffle the clinician as much as it confuses the student. A colossal volume of literature on understanding ECG bears testimony to this fact. Yet mastering the ECG remains a formidable task and an elusive dream.

The present book is another attempt to bring the subject of ECG closer to the hearts of students and clinicians, but with a difference. As the book unfolds, the subject gradually evolves from basics to therapeutics. Although emphasis is on ECG appearances, causation of abnormalities and their clinical relevance are briefly mentioned. This should help students preparing for their examinations as they would not have to refer to voluminous textbooks.

Some arrhythmias are harmless, others are ominous and a few require resuscitation. The real challenge lies in knowing the cause of an arrhythmia, its clinical significance, differential diagnosis and practical aspects of management. Therefore, seemingly similar cardiac rhythms are discussed together under one chapter heading. Medical students, resident doctors, nurses and technicians will find this format particularly useful.

I have thoroughly enjoyed the experience of writing this book and found teaching as pleasurable as learning. Since the scope for further refinement and improvement always remians, it is a privilege to bring out the 3rd edition of ECG Made Easy. Your appreciation, encouragement, comments and criticisms and bound to spur me on into the future.

Atul Luthra

ACKNOWLEDGEMENTS

I am extremely grateful to:

- My school teachers who helped me to acquire good command over the English language.
- My professors at medical college who taught me the science and art of clinical medicine.
- My heart patients whose cardiograms stimulated my grey matter to write a book
- Authors of texts on electrocardiography to which I referred liberally while preparing the manuscript.
- M/s Jaypee Brothers Medical Publishers (P) Ltd who reposed their faith in me and provided encouragement, expert counseling and editorial assistance.
- My readers whose generous appreciation, candid comments and constructive criticism spur me on to improve further.

CONTENTS

CHAPTER 1

Nomenclature of ECG Deflections, Intervals and Segments

THE ELECTROCARDIOGRAM (ECG)

The electrocardiogram provides a graphic depiction of the electrical forces generated by the heart. The ECG graph appears as a series of deflections and waves produced by each cardiac cycle.

Before going on to the genesis of individual deflections and their terminology, it would be worthwhile mentioning certain important facts about the direction and magnitude of ECG waves and the activation pattern of myocardium.

Direction

- By convention, a deflection above the baseline or iso-electric (neutral) line is a positive deflection while one below the isoelectric line is a negative deflection (Fig. 1.1).

  The direction of a deflection depends upon two factors namely, the direction of spread of the electrical force and the location of the recording electrode.

  In other words, an electrical impulse moving towards an electrode creates a positive deflection while an impulse moving away from an electrode creates a negative deflection (Fig. 1.1). Let us see this example.

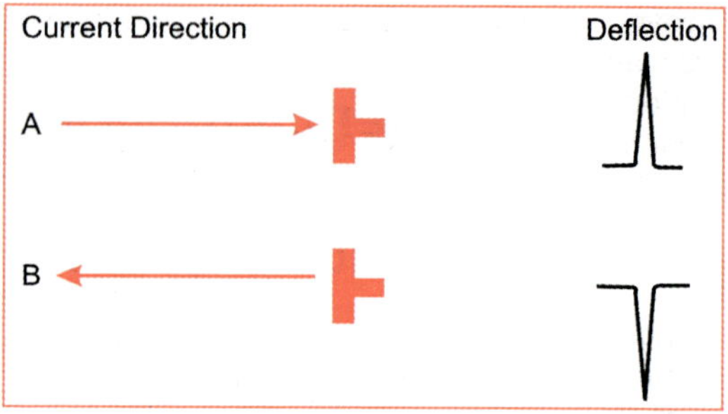

Fig. 1.1: Effect of current direction on polarity of ECG deflection
A. Towards the electrode—positive/upright deflection
B. Away from electrode—negative/inverted deflection

We know that the sequence of electrical activation is such that the interventricular septum is first activated from left to right followed by activation of the left ventricular free wall from the endocardial to epicardial surface.

If an electrode is placed over the right ventricle, it records an initial positive deflection representing septal activation towards it, followed by a major negative deflection that denotes free wall activation away from it (Fig. 1.2).

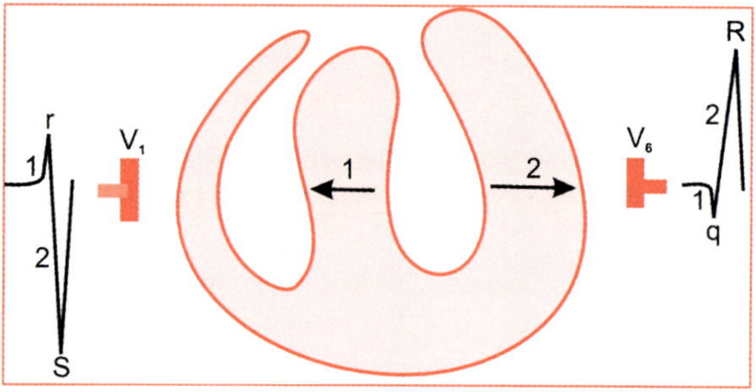

Fig. 1.2: Septal (1) and left ventricular (2) activation viewed from lead V_1 (rS pattern) and lead V_6 (qR pattern)

If however, the electrode is placed over the left ventricle, it records an initial negative deflection representing septal activation away from it, followed by a major positive deflection that denotes free wall activation towards it (Fig. 1.2).

Magnitude

- The magnitude of a deflection depends upon the quantum of the electrical forces generated by the heart and the extent to which they are transmitted to the recording electrode on the body surface. Let us see these examples:

  Since the ventricle has a far greater muscle mass than the atrium, ventricular complexes are larger than atrial complexes.

  When the ventricular wall undergoes thickening (hypertrophy), the ventricular complexes are larger than normal.

  If the chest wall is thick, the ventricular complexes are smaller than normal since the fat or muscle intervenes between the myocardium and the recording electrode (Fig. 1.3).

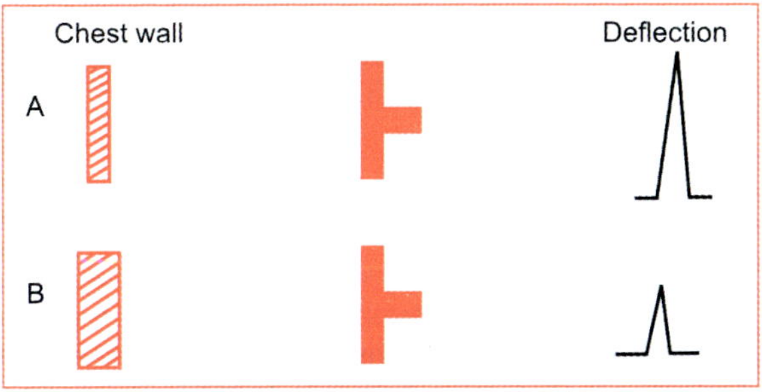

Fig. 1.3: Effect of chest wall thickness on magnitude of deflection
A. Thin chest—tall deflection
B. Thick chest—small deflection

Activation

- Activation of the atria occurs longitudinally by contiguous spread of electrical forces from one muscle fibre to the other. On the other hand, activation of the ventricles occurs transversely by spread of electrical forces from the endocardial surface (surface facing ventricular cavity) to the epicardial surface (outer surface) (Fig. 1.4).

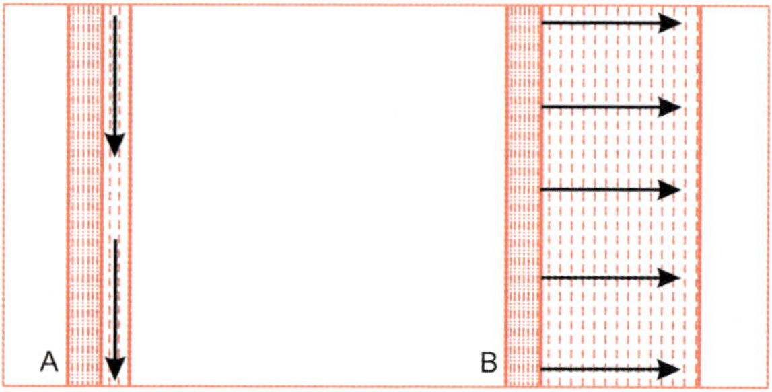

Fig. 1.4: Direction of myocardial activation in atrium and ventricle
A. Atrial—longitudinal, from one fibre to other fibre
B. Ventricular—transverse, endocardium to epicardium

Therefore, atrial activation can reflect atrial enlargement (and not atrial hypertrophy) while ventricular activation can reflect ventricular hypertrophy (and not ventricular enlargement).

THE ELECTROPHYSIOLOGY

The ECG graph consists of a series of deflections or waves. The distances between sequential waves on the time axis are termed as intervals. Portions of the isoelectric line (baseline) between successive waves are termed as segments.

In order to understand the genesis of deflections and the significance of intervals and segments, it would be worthwhile understanding certain basic electrophysiological principles.

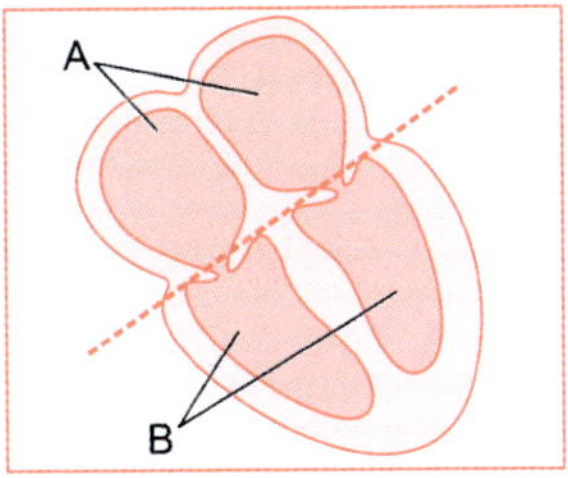

Fig. 1.5: The "dual-chamber" concept
A. Biatrial chamber
B. Biventricular chamber

- Anatomically speaking, the heart is a four-chambered organ. But in the electrophysiological sense, it is actually two-chambered. As per the "dual-chamber" concept, the chambers of the heart are the bi-atrial chamber and the bi-ventricular chamber (Fig. 1.5).

  This is because the atria are activated together and the ventricles too contact synchronously. Therefore, on the ECG, atrial activation is represented by a single wave and ventricular activation by a single wave-complex.

- In the resting state, the muscle cell membrane bears a negative charge on the inside. When stimulated by an electrical impulse, the charge is altered by a shift of electrolytes (sodium and calcium) across the cell membrane.

  This results in coupling of actin and myosin filaments and muscle contraction. The spread of electrical impulse through the myocardium is known as depolarization (Fig. 1.6).

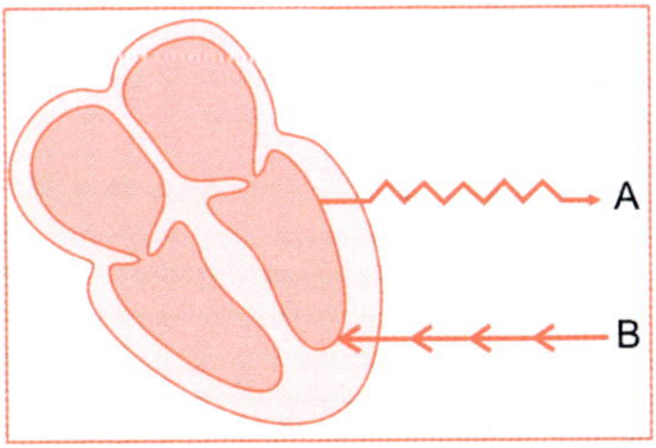

Fig. 1.6: The spread of impulse
A. Depolarization
B. Repolarization

Once the muscle contraction is completed, there is once again a shift of electrolytes, in order to restore the resting state of the cell membrane. This results in uncoupling of actin and myosin filaments and muscle relaxation. The return of the myocardium to its resting electrical state is known as repolarization (Fig. 1.6).

Depolarization and repolarization occur in the atrial muscle as well as in the ventricular myocardium. The wave of excitation is synchronised so that the atria and the ventricles contract and relax in a rhythmic sequence.

Atrial depolarization is followed by atrial repolarization which is nearly synchronous with ventricular depolarization and finally ventricular repolarization occurs.

We must appreciate that depolarization and repolarization of the heart muscle are electrical events, while cardiac contraction (systole) and relaxation (diastole) constitute mechanical events.

However, it is true that depolarization just precedes systole and repolarization is immediately followed by diastole.

- The electrical impulse that initiates myocardial depolarization and contraction originates from a group of cells that comprise the pacemaker of the heart.

The normal pacemaker is the sinoatrial (SA) node, situated in the upper portion of the right atrium (Fig. 1.7).

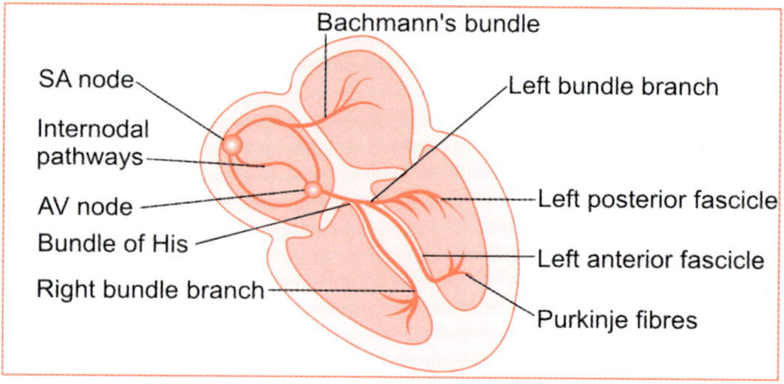

Fig. 1.7: The electrical 'wiring' network of the heart

From the SA node, the electrical impulse spreads to the right atrium through three intra-atrial pathways while the Bachmann's bundle carries the impulse to the left atrium.

Having activated the atria, the impulse enters the atrioventricular (AV) node situated at the AV junction, on the lower part of the inter-atrial septum. The brief delay of the impulse at the AV node allows time for the atria to empty the blood they contain into their respective ventricles.

After the AV nodal delay, the impulse travels to the ventricles through a specialized conduction system called the bundle of His. The His bundle primarily divides into two branches, a right bundle branch (RBB) which traverses the right ventricle and a left bundle branch (LBB) that traverses the left ventricle (Fig. 1.7).

A small septal branch originates from the left bundle branch to activate the interventricular septum from left to right. The left bundle branch further divides into a left posterior fascicle and a left anterior fascicle.

The posterior fascicle is a broad band of fibres which spreads over the posterior and inferior surfaces of the left ventricle. The anterior fascicle is a narrow band of fibres which spreads over the anterior and superior surfaces of the left ventricle (Fig. 1.7).

Having transversed the bundle branches, the impulse finally passes into their terminal ramifications called Purkinje fibres. These Purkinje fibres traverse the thickness of the myocardium to activate the entire myocardial mass from the endocardial surface to the epicardial surface.

THE DEFLECTIONS

The ECG graph consists of a series of deflections or waves. Each electrocardiographic deflection has been arbitrarily assigned a letter of the alphabet. Accordingly, a sequence of

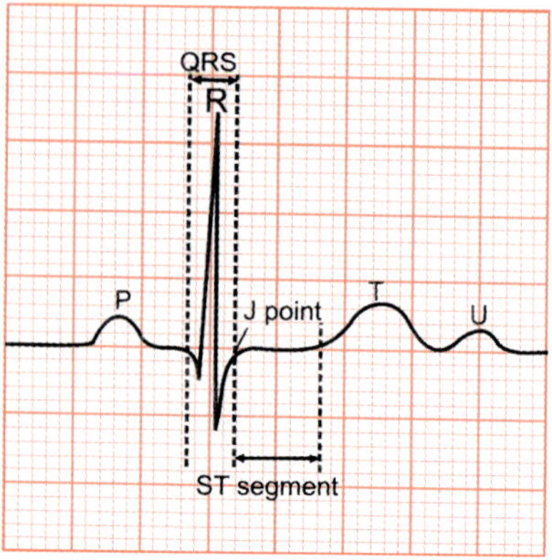

Fig. 1.8: The normal ECG deflections

wave that represents a single cardiac cycle is sequentially termed as P Q R S T and U (Fig. 1.8).

By convention, P, T and U waves are always denoted by capital letters while the Q, R and S waves can be represented by either a capital letter or a small letter depending upon their relative or absolute magnitude. Large waves (over 5 mm) are assigned capital letters Q, R and S while small waves (under 5 mm) are assigned small letters q, r and s.

Relatively speaking, a small q followed by a tall R is labelled as qR complex while a large Q followed by a small r is labelled as Qr complex. Similarly, a small r followed by a deep S is termed as rS complex while a tall R followed by a small s is termed as Rs complex (Fig. 1.9).

Two other situations are worth mentioning. If a QRS deflection is totally negative without an ensuing positivity, it is termed as a QS complex.

Secondly, if the QRS complex reflects two positive waves, the second positive wave is termed as R' and accordingly, the complex is termed as rSR' or RsR' depending upon magnitude of the positive (r or R) wave and the negative (s or S) wave (Fig. 1.9).

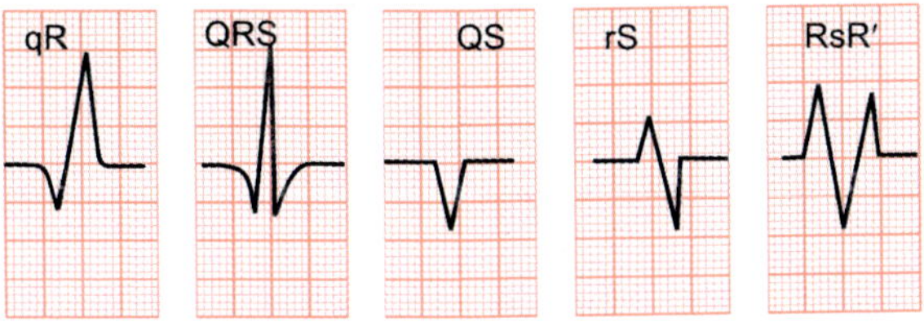

Fig. 1.9: Various configurations of the QRS complex

Significance of ECG Deflections

P wave	:	Produced by atrial depolarization.
QRS complex	:	Produced by ventricular depolarization. It consists of:
Q wave	:	First negative deflection before R wave.
R wave	:	First positive deflection after Q wave.
S wave	:	First negative deflection after R wave.
T wave	:	Produced by ventricular repolarization.
U wave	:	Produced by Purkinje system repolarization (Fig. 1.10).

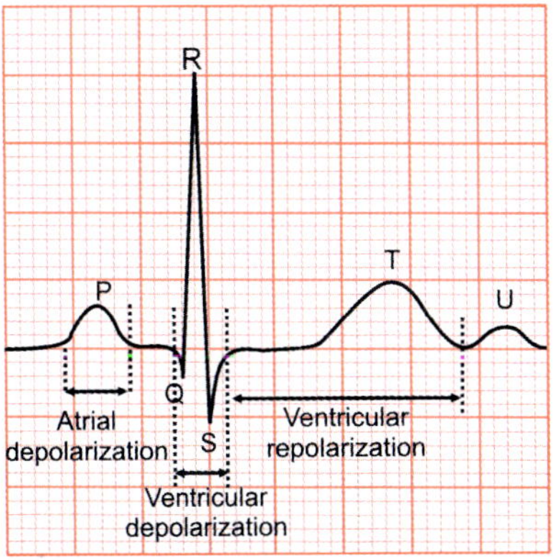

Fig. 1.10: Depolarization and repolarization depicted as deflections. (Note: Atrial repolarization is buried in the QRS complex)

You would be wondering where is atrial repolarization. Well, it is represented by the Ta wave which occurs after the P wave. The Ta wave is actually not seen on the ECG as it coincides with (buried in) the larger QRS complex.

THE INTERVALS

During analysis of an ECG graph, the distances between certain waves are relevant in order to establish a temporal relationship between sequential events during a cardiac cycle. Since the distance between waves is expressed on a time axis, these distances are termed as ECG intervals. The following ECG intervals are clinically important.

P-R Interval

The P-R interval is measured from the onset of the P wave to the beginning of the QRS complex (Fig. 1.11). Although the term P-R interval is in vogue, actually, P-Q interval would be more appropriate. Note that the duration of the P wave is included in the measurement.

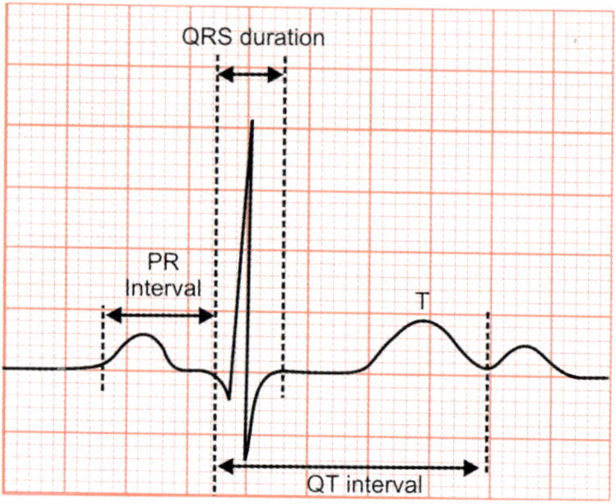

Fig. 1.11: The normal ECG intervals

We know that the P wave represents atrial depolarization while the QRS complex represents ventricular depolarization. Therefore, it is easy to comprehend that the P-R interval is an expression of atrioventricular conduction time.

This includes the time for atrial depolarization, conduction delay in the AV node and the time required for the impulse to transverse the ventricular conduction system before ventricular depolarization ensues.

Q-T Interval

The Q-T interval is measured from the onset of the Q wave to the end of the T wave (Fig. 1.11). If it is measured to the end of the U wave, it is termed Q-U interval. Note that the duration of the QRS complex, the length of the ST segment and the duration of the T wave are included in the measurement.

We know that the QRS complex represents ventricular depolarization while the T wave represents ventricular repolarization. Therefore, it is easy to comprehend that the Q-T interval is an expression of total duration of ventricular systole.

Since the U wave represents Purkinje system repolarization, the Q-U interval in addition, takes into account the time taken for the ventricular Purkinje system to repolarize.

THE SEGMENTS

The magnitude and direction of an ECG deflection is expressed in relation to a base-line which is referred to as the isoelectric line. The main isoelectric line is the period of electrical inactivity that intervenes between successive cardiac cycles during which no deflections are observed.

It lies between the termination of the T wave (or U wave if seen) of one cardiac cycle and onset of the P wave of the next cardiac cycle. However, two other segments of the isoelectric line, that occur between the waves of a single cardiac cycle, are clinically important.

P-R Segment

The P-R segment is that portion of the isoelectric line which intervenes between the termination of the P wave and the onset of the QRS complex (Fig. 1.12). Note carefully that the length of the P-R segment does not include the width of the P wave while the duration of the P-R interval does include the P wave width.

S-T Segment

The S-T segment is that portion of the isoelectric line which intervenes between the termination of the S wave and the onset of the T wave (Fig. 1.12). The point at which the QRS complex ends and the ST segment begins is termed the junction point or J point.

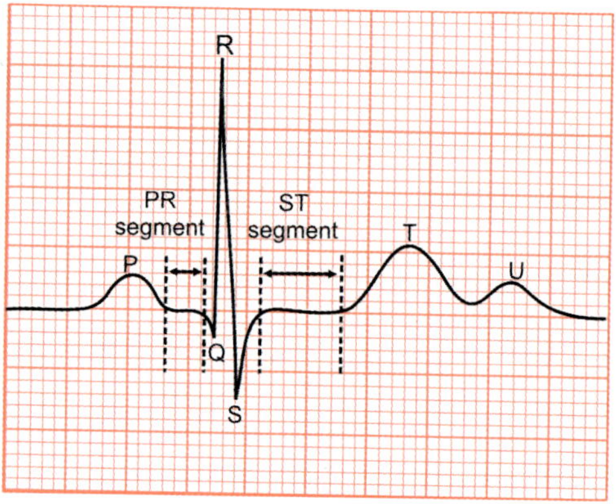

Fig. 1.12: The normal ECG segments

CHAPTER 2

The Electrocardiographic Leads

THE ELECTROCARDIOGRAPHIC LEADS

During activation of the myocardium, electrical forces or action potentials are propagated in various directions. These electrical forces can be picked up from the surface of the body by means of electrodes and recorded in the form of an electrocardiogram.

A pair of electrodes, that consists of a positive and a negative electrode constitutes an electrocardiographic lead. Each lead is oriented to record electrical forces as viewed from one aspect of the heart.

The position of these electrodes can be changed so that different leads are obtained. The angle of electrical activity recorded changes with each lead. Several angles of recording provide a detailed perspective the heart.

There are twelve conventional ECG lead placements that constitute the routine 12-lead ECG (Fig. 2.1).

The 12 ECG leads are:

- Limb leads or extremity leads—six in number.
- Chest leads or precordial leads—six in number

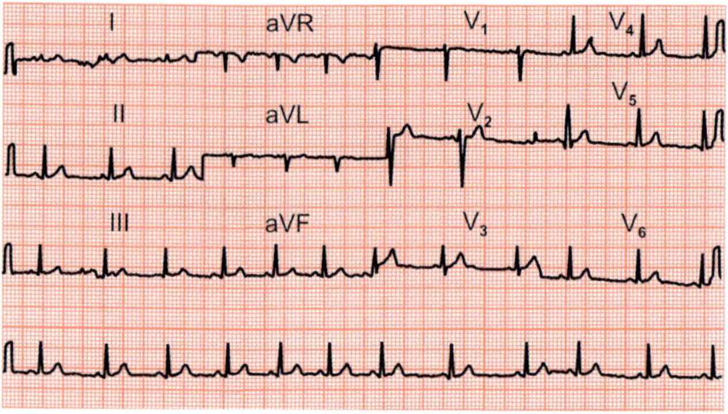

Fig. 2.1: The conventional 12-lead electrocardiogram

THE LIMB LEADS

The limb leads are derived from electrodes placed on the limbs. An electrode is placed on each of the three limbs namely right arm, left arm and left leg. The right leg electrode acts as the grounding electrode (Fig. 2.2A).

- Standard limb leads—three in number.
- Augmented limb leads—three in number.

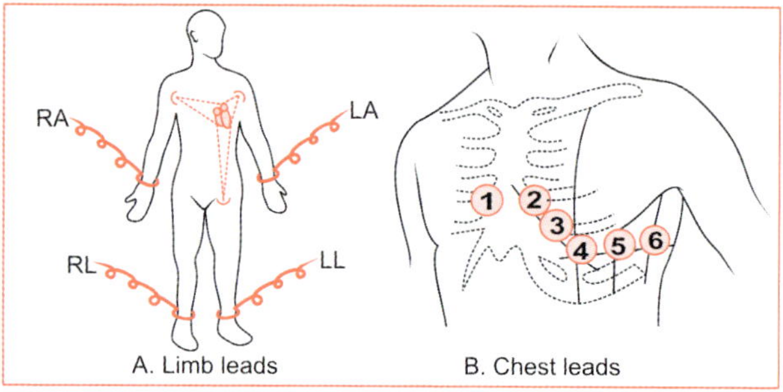

Fig. 2.2: Electrode placement for ECG recording

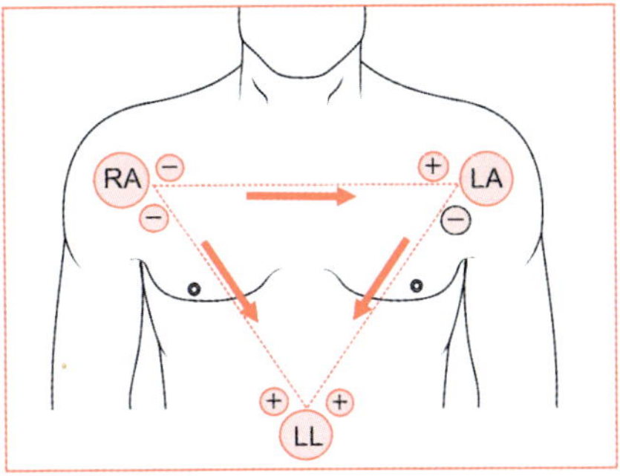

Fig. 2.3: The three standard limb leads: L_I, L_{II} and L_{III}

Standard Limb Leads

The standard limb leads obtain a graph of the electrical forces as recorded between two limbs at a time. Therefore, the standard limb leads are also called bipolar leads. In these leads, on limb carries a positive electrode and the other limb carries a negative electrode. There are three standard limb leads (Fig. 2.3):

- Lead L_I
- Lead L_{II}
- Lead L_{III}

Lead	*Positive electrode*	*Negative electrode*
I	LA	RA
II	LL	RA
III	LL	LA

Augmented Limb Leads

The augmented limb leads obtain a graph of the electrical forces as recorded from one limb at a time. Therefore, the augmented limb leads are also called unipolar leads. In these

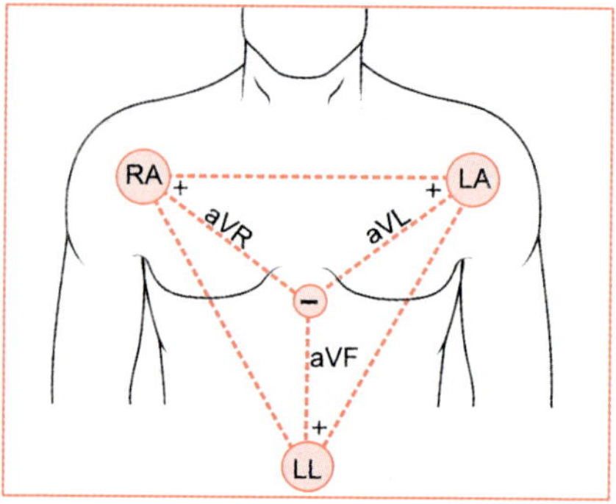

Fig. 2.4: The three unipolar limb leads: aVR, aVL and aVF

leads, one limb carries a positive electrode, while a central terminal represents the negative pole which is actually at zero potential. There are three augmented limb leads (Fig. 2.4):

- Lead aVR (Right arm)
- Lead aVL (Left arm)
- Lead aVF (Foot left)

Lead	*Positive electrode*
aVR	RA
aVL	LA
aVF	LL

THE CHEST LEADS

The chest leads are obtained from electrodes placed on the precordium in designated areas. An electrode can be placed on six different positions on the left side of the chest, each position representing one lead (Fig. 2.2B). Accordingly, there are six chest leads namely:

- Lead V_1 : Over the fourth intercostal space, just to the right of sternal border.

- Lead V_2 : Over the fourth intercostal space, just to the left of sternal border.
- Lead V_3 : Over a point midway between V_2 and V_4 (see V_4 below).
- Lead V_4 : Over the fifth intercostal space in the midclavicular line.
- Lead V_5 : Over the anterior axillary line, at the same level as lead V_4.
- Lead V_6 : Over the midaxillary line, at the same level as leads V_4 and V_5.

Sometimes, the chest leads are obtained from electrodes placed on the right side of the chest. The right-sided chest leads are V_{1R}, V_{2R}, V_{3R}, V_{4R}, V_{5R} and V_{6R}. These leads are mirror-images of the standard left-sided chest leads.

V_{1R} : 4th intercostal space to left of sternum

V_{2R} : 4th intercostal space to right of sternum

V_{3R} : Point mid-way between V_{2R} and V_{4R}

V_{4R} : 5th intercostal space in midclavicular line, and so on.

The right-sided chest leads are particularly useful for the assessment of the right ventricle.

THE LEAD ORIENTATION

We have thus seen that the 12-lead ECG consists of the following 12 leads recorded in succession:

L_I L_{II} L_{III} aVR aVL aVF V_1 V_2 V_3 V_4 V_5 V_6

Since the left ventricle is the dominant and clinically the most important chamber of the heart, it needs to be assessed in detail. The left ventricle can be viewed from different angles, each with a specific set of leads. The leads with respect to different regions of the left ventricle, are shown in Table 2.1.

Table 2.1: Region of left ventricle represented on ECG

ECG leads	*Region of left ventricle*
V_1, V_2	Septal
V_3, V_4	Anterior
V_5, V_6	Lateral
V_1 to V_4	Antero-septal
V_3 to V_6	Antero-lateral
L_I, aVL	High lateral
L_{II}, L_{III}, aVF	Inferior

THE EINTHOVEN TRIANGLE

We have seen that the standard limb leads are recorded from two limbs at a time, one carrying the positive electrode and the other, the negative electrode. The three standard limb leads (L_I, L_{II}, L_{III}) can be seen to form an equilateral triangle with the heart at the centre. This triangle is called the *Einthoven triangle* (Fig. 2.5A).

To facilitate the graphic representation of electrical forces, the three limbs of the Einthoven triangle can be redrawn in such a way that the three leads they represent bisect each other and

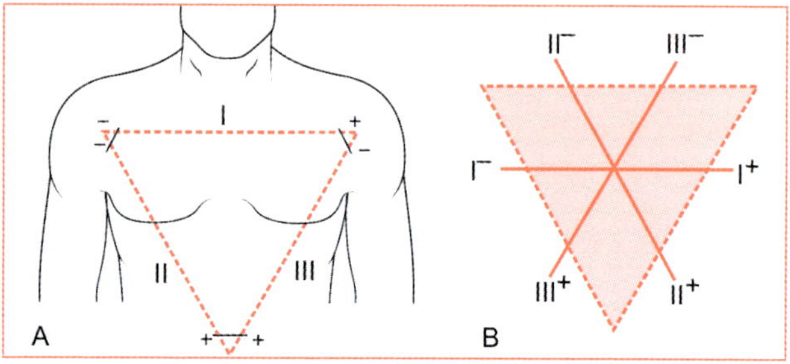

Fig. 2.5: A. The Einthoven triangle of limb leads
B. The triaxial reference system

pass through a common central point. This produces a triaxial reference system with each axis separated by 60° from the other, the lead polarity (+ or –) and direction remaining the same (Fig. 2.5B).

We have also seen that the augmented limb leads are recorded from one limb at a time, the limb carrying the positive electrode and the negative pole being represented by the central point. The three augmented limb leads (aVR, aVL, aVF) can be seen to form another triaxial reference system with each axis being separated by 60° from one other (Fig. 2.6A).

When this triaxial system of unipolar leads is superimposed on the triaxial system of limb leads, we can derive a hexaxial reference system with each axis being separated by 30° from the other (Fig. 2.6B).

Note carefully that each of the six leads retains its polarity (positive and negative poles) and orientation (lead direction).

The hexaxial reference system concept is important in determining the major direction of the heart's electrical forces. As we shall see later, this is what we call the electrical axis of the QRS complex.

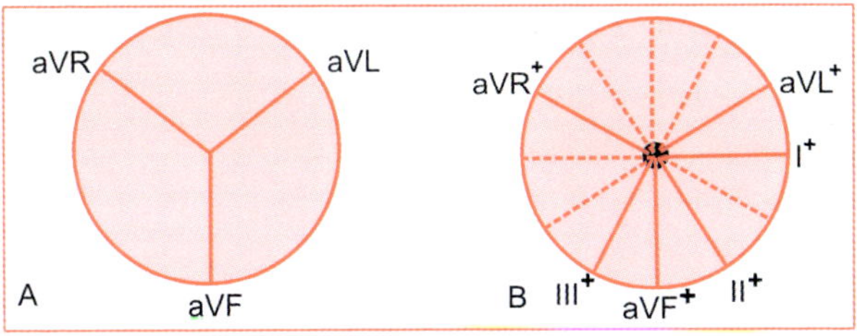

Fig. 2.6: A. The triaxial reference system from unipolar leads
B. The hexaxial system from unipolar and limb leads

CHAPTER 3

The ECG Grid and Normal Values

THE ECG GRID

The electrocardiography paper is made in such a way that it is thermosensitive. Therefore, the ECG is recorded by movement of the tip of a heated stylus over the moving paper.

The ECG paper is available as a roll of 20 or 30 metres which when loaded into the ECG machine moves at a predetermined speed of 25 mm per second.

The ECG paper is marked like a graph, consisting of horizontal and vertical lines. There are fine lines marked 1 mm apart while every fifth line in marked boldly. Therefore, the bold lines are placed 5 mm apart (Fig. 3.1).

Time is measured along the horizontal axis in seconds while voltage is measured along the vertical axis in millivolts.

During ECG recording, the usual paper speed is 25 mm per second. This means that 25 small squares are covered in one second. In other words, the width of 1 small square is 1/25 or 0.04 seconds and the width of 1 large square is 0.04 × 5 or 0.2 seconds.

Therefore, the width of an ECG deflection or the duration of an ECG interval is the number of small squares it occupies on the horizontal axis multiplied by 0.04 (Fig. 3.1). Accordingly, 2 small

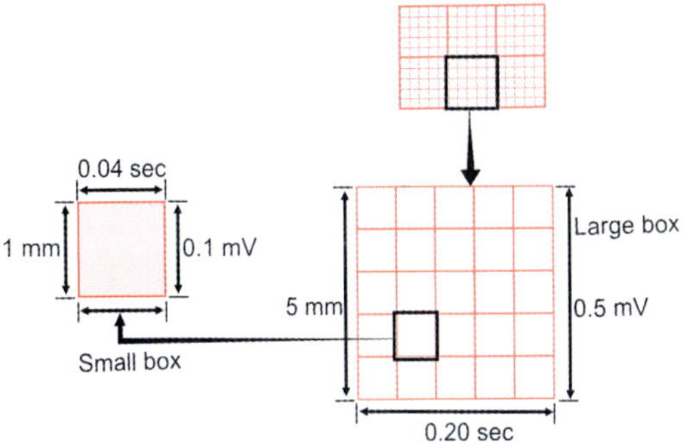

Fig. 3.1: The enlarged illustration of the electrocardiography paper
1 small square = 1 mm. 5 small squares = 1 big square
Vertically, 1 small square = 0.1 mV. 5 of them = 0.5 mV
Horizontally, 1 small square = 0.04 sec. 5 of them = 0.2 sec

squares represent 0.08 sec., 3 small squares represent 0.12 sec. and 6 small squares represent 0.24 sec.

Normally, the ECG machine is standardised in such a way that a 1 millivolt signal from the machine produces a 10 millimetre vertical deflection. In other words, each small square on the vertical axis represents 0.1 mV and each large square represents 0.5 mV.

Therefore, the height of a positive deflection (above the base-line) or the depth of a negative deflection (below the base-line) is the number of small squares it occupies on the vertical axis multiplied by 0.1 mV (Fig. 3.1). Accordingly, 3 small squares represent 0.3 mV, 1 large square represents 0.5 mV and 6 small squares represent 0.6 mV.

Similarly, the degree of elevation (above the base-line) or depression (below the base-line) of segment is expressed in number of small squares (millimetres) of segment elevation or segment depression, in relation to the isoelectric line.

THE NORMAL ECG VALUES

Normal P Wave

The P wave is a small rounded wave produced by atrial depolarization. In fact, it reflects the sum of right and left atrial activation, the right preceding the left since the pacemaker is located in the right atrium (Fig. 3.2A).

The P wave is normally upright in most of the ECG leads with two exceptions. In lead aVR, it is inverted along with inversion of the QRS complex and the T wave, since the direction of atrial activation is away from this lead.

In lead V_1, it is generally biphasic that is, upright but with a small terminal negative deflection, representing left atrial activation in a reverse direction.

Normally, the P wave has a single peak without a gap or notch between the right and left atrial components. A normal P wave meets the following criteria:

- Less than 2.5 mm (0.25 mV) in height
- Less than 2.5 mm (0.10 sec) in width (Fig. 3.2B)

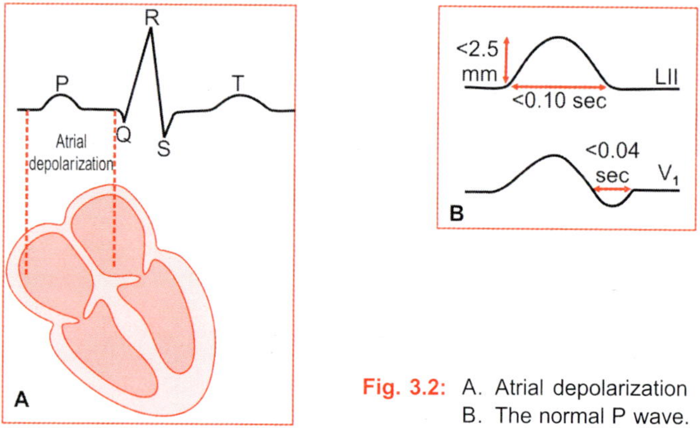

Fig. 3.2: A. Atrial depolarization
B. The normal P wave.

Normal QRS Complex

The QRS complex is the major positive deflection on the ECG produced by ventricular depolarization. In fact, it represents the timing and sequence of synchronised depolarization of the right and left ventricles.

The Q wave is not visible in all ECG leads. Physiological Q waves may be observed in leads L_I, aVL, V_5 and V_6 where they represent initial activation of the interventricular septum in a direction opposite to the direction of activation of the main left ventricular mass.

A physiological Q wave meets the following criteria:

- Less than 0.04 sec in width
- Less than 25 percent of R wave (Fig. 3.3A).

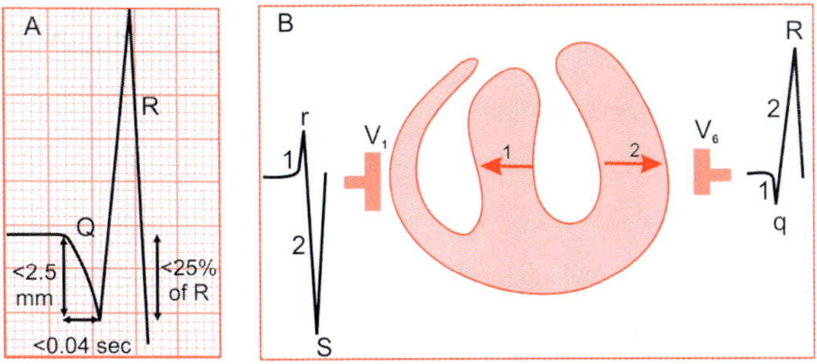

Fig. 3.3: A. The normal Q wave. B. Septal depolarization

The leads in which physiological Q waves appear depends upon the direction towards which the main mass of the left ventricle is oriented.

If the left ventricle is directed towards the lateral leads (horizontal heart), Q waves appear in leads L_I, aVL, V_5 and V_6 (Fig. 3.3B). If it is directed towards the inferior leads (vertical heart), Q waves appear in leads L_{II}, L_{III} and aVF.

The R wave is the major positive deflection of the QRS complex. It is upright in most leads except in lead aVR where the P wave and T wave are also inverted.

In the limb leads, R wave voltage is normally atleast 5 mm while in the precordial leads, R wave voltage exceeds 10 mm.

Under normal circumstances, the R wave voltage gradually increases as we move from lead V_1 to lead V_6. This is known as normal R wave progression in precordial leads.

Normally, the R wave amplitude does not exceed 0.4 mV (4 mm) in lead V_1 where it reflects septal activation and does not exceed 2.5 mV (25 mm) in lead V_6 where it reflects left ventricular activation (Fig. 3.4A).

The r wave is smaller than the S wave in lead V_1 and the R wave is taller than the s wave in lead V_6.

The S wave is the negative deflection that follows the R wave, representing the terminal portion of ventricular depolarization.

In lead V_1, the S wave reflects left ventricular activation while in lead V_6 the s wave reflects right ventricular activation.

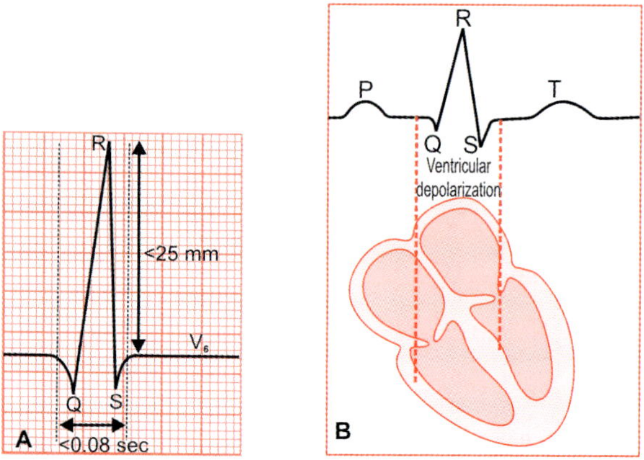

Fig. 3.4: A. The normal QRS complex. B. Ventricular depolarization

Normally, the S wave magnitude is greater than the r wave height in lead V_1 and the s wave is smaller than the R wave in lead V_6. The normal s wave voltage in lead V_6 does not exceed 0.7 mV.

The QRS complex represents depolarization of the total ventricular muscle. The relative amplitude of the R wave and S wave in a particular lead reflects the relative contributions of the right and left ventricles.

For instance in lead V_1, the r wave is smaller than the S wave while in lead V_6 the s wave is smaller than the R wave.

The duration of the QRS complex is the total time taken for both ventricles to be depolarized. Since the right and left ventricles are depolarized in a synchronous fashion, the normal QRS complex is narrow, has a sharp peak and measures less than 0.08 sec (2 mm) on the horizontal axis (Fig. 3.4B).

Normal T Wave

The T wave is a large rounded wave produced by ventricular repolarization (Fig. 3.5). The T wave is normally upright in most leads with certain exceptions.

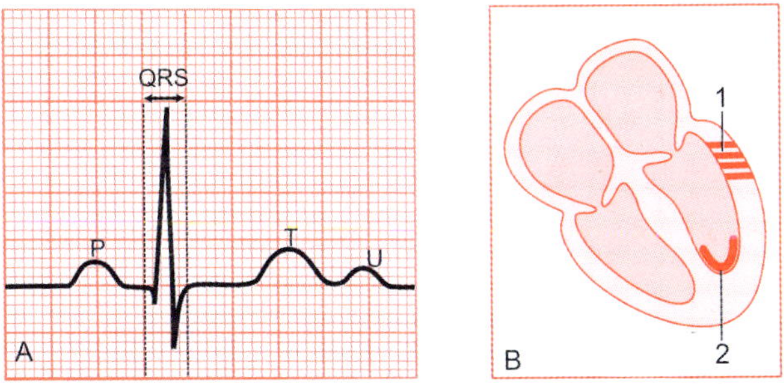

Fig. 3.5: A. The normal T and U waves.
B. T wave (1): ventricular mass repolarization,
U wave (2): Purkinje system repolarization

It is invariably inverted in lead aVR along with inversion of the P wave and QRS complex. It is often inverted in lead V_1, occasionally in lead V_2 V_3 and sometimes in lead L_{III}.

The normal T wave is taller in lead V_6 than in lead V_1. The amplitude of the normal T wave does not generally exceed 5 mm in the limb leads and 10 mm in the precordial leads.

Normal U Wave

The U wave is a small rounded wave produced by slow and late repolarization of the intraventricular Purkinje system, after the main ventricular mass has been repolarized (Fig. 3.5).

It is often difficult to notice the U wave but when seen, it is best appreciated in the precordial leads V_2 to V_4. The U wave is more easy to recognise when the Q-T interval is short or the heart rate is slow, in which conditions it is clearly separated from the preceding T wave and the P wave of the following beat, respectively.

The normal U wave is upright and it is normally much smaller than the T wave which it follows.

Normal P-R Interval

The P-R interval is measured on the horizontal axis from the onset of the P wave to the beginning of the QRS complex, irrespective of whether it begins with a Q wave or a R wave (Fig. 3.6).

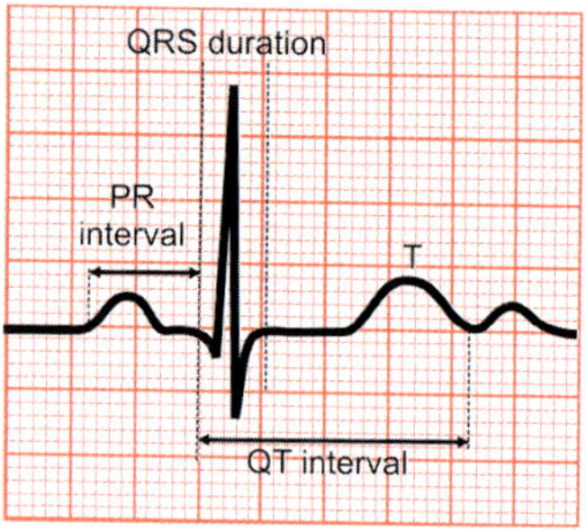

Fig. 3.6: The normal ECG intervals

Since the P wave represents atrial depolarization and the QRS complex represents ventricular depolarization, the P-R interval is a measure of the atrioventricular (AV) conduction time.

The A-V conduction time includes time for atrial depolarization, conduction delay in the AV node and time required for the impulse to traverse the conduction system before ventricular depolarization begins.

The normal P-R interval is in the range of 0.12 to 0.20 sec, depending upon the heart rate. It is prolonged at slow heart rates and shortened at fast heart rates. The P-R interval tends to be slightly shorter in children (upper limit 0.18 sec) and slightly longer in elderly persons (upper limit 0.22 sec).

Normal Q-T Interval

The Q-T interval is measured on the horizontal axis from the onset of the Q wave to the end of the T wave (Fig. 3.6).

Since the QRS complex represents ventricular depolarization and the T wave represents ventricular repolarization, Q-T interval denotes the total duration of ventricular systole.

The Q-T interval includes the duration of QRS complex, the length of S-T segment and the width of the T wave.

The normal Q-T interval is in the range of 0.35 to 0.43 sec or 0.39 $\pm$ 0.04 sec. The Q-T interval depends upon three variables namely age, sex and heart rate.

The Q-T interval tends to be shorter in young individuals and longer in the elderly. It is normally, slightly shorter in females, the upper limit being 0.42 sec. The Q-T interval shortens at fast heart rates and lengthens at slow heart rates.

Therefore, for proper interpretation, the Q-T interval must be corrected for the heart rate. The corrected Q-T interval is known as the Q-Tc interval. The Q-Tc interval is determined using the formula:

$$\text{Q - Tc} = \frac{\text{Q - T}}{\sqrt{\text{R-R}}}$$

where, Q-T is the measured Q-T interval, and

$\sqrt{\text{R-R}}$ is the square-root of the measured R-R interval.

Since, the R-R interval at a heart rate of 60 is 25 mm or 1 second (25 × 0.04 sec = 1 sec), the Q-Tc interval is equal to the Q-T interval at a heart rate of 60 per minute.

Normal P-R Segment

That portion of the baseline (isoelectric line) which intervenes between the termination of the P wave and the onset of the QRS complex, is the P-R segment (Fig. 3.7).

Normally, it is at level with the main segment of the isoelectric line which intervenes between the T wave of one cycle and the P wave of the next cycle.

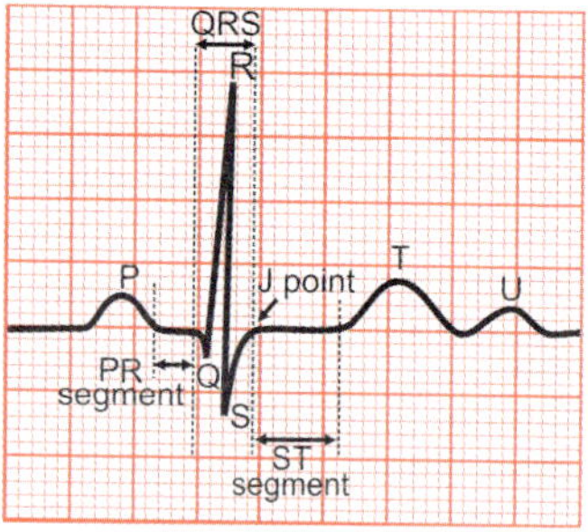

Fig. 3.7: The normal ECG segments

Normal S-T Segment

That portion of the baseline (isoelectric line) which intervenes between the termination of the S wave and the onset of the T wave, is the S-T segment (Fig. 3.7).

The beginning of the S-T segment is the junction point (J point). Normally, the S-T segment and the J point are in level with the main segment of the isoelectric line which intervenes between the T wave of one cycle and the P wave of the next cycle.

CHAPTER 4 Determination of the Electrical Axis

THE ELECTRICAL AXIS

During activation of the heart, the electrical forces or action potentials which have been generated, are propagated in various directions. These electrical forces can be picked up from the surface of the body by means of electrodes.

Normally, over 80 percent of these forces are cancelled out by equal and opposing forces, and only the net forces remaining are recorded. The dominant direction of these forces, which is the mean of all recorded forces, constitutes the electrical axis of an electrocardiographic deflection.

Since the QRS complex is the major deflection on the ECG, we shall confine ourselves to the QRS electrical axis.

THE HEXAXIAL SYSTEM

We have already seen that the three standard limb leads L_I, L_{II} and L_{III} form an equilateral triangle with the heart at its centre, which is called the Einthoven triangle.

The Einthoven triangle can be redrawn in such a way that the three leads pass through a common central point. This constitutes a triaxial reference system with each axis separated from the other by 60°.

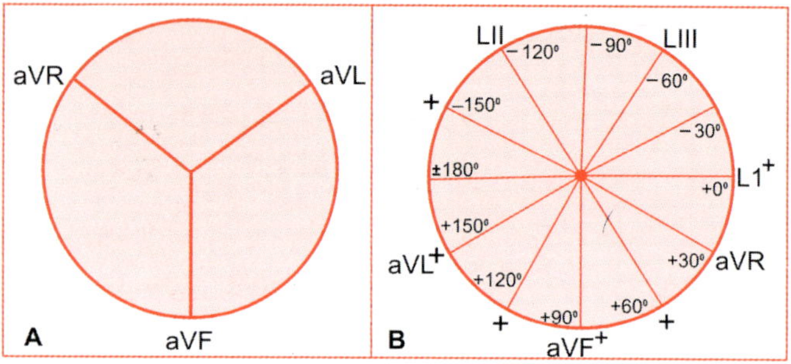

Fig. 4.1: A. The triaxial reference system from unipolar leads
B. The hexaxial system from unipolar and limb leads

Similarly, the three augmented limb leads can constitute another triaxial reference system (Fig. 4.1A). When these two triaxial systems are superimposed on each other, we can derive a hexaxial reference system in a 360° circle, with each axis separated from the other by 30° (Fig. 4.1B).

In the hexaxial system, each of the six leads maintains its own polarity and direction. The hexaxial reference system is the basis of understanding the concept of electrical axis and its determination.

THE QRS AXIS

Before going on to the actual determination of the QRS axis, certain basic principles have to be understood.

- The QRS axis is expressed as a degree on the hexaxial system and represents the direction of electrical forces in the frontal plane (Fig. 4.2).
- The net deflection in any lead is the algebraic sum of the positive and negative deflections. For instance, if in any lead the positive deflection (R) is +6 and the negative deflection (S) is –2, the net deflection is +4.

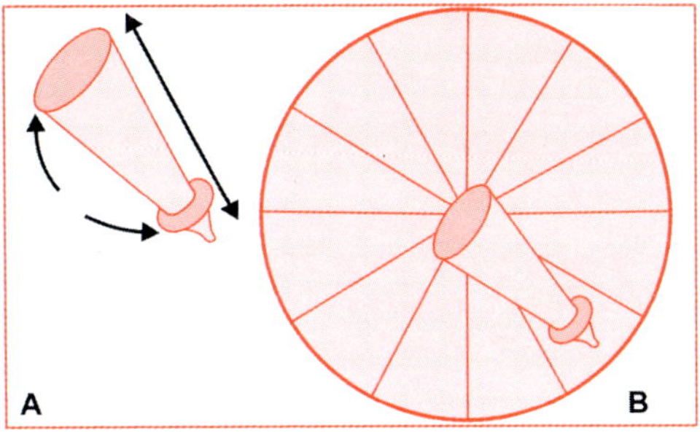

Fig. 4.2: A. The direction and magnitude of the QRS vector
B. The QRS vector projected on the hexaxial system

- An electrical force that runs parallel to any lead, records the maximum deflection in that lead. An electrical force that runs obliquely to any lead, records a small deflection in that lead. An electrical force that runs perpendicular to any lead records a nil or equiphasic (positive and negative deflections equal) deflection in that lead.
- For instance, if the axis is +90°, lead aVF records the maximum deflection. Lead L_I records the least deflection and the deflections in all other leads are intermediate.
- If in the lead showing the maximum deflection, the major deflection is positive, the axis points towards the positive pole of that lead. Conversely, if the major deflection is negative, the axis points towards the negative pole of that particular lead.
- For instance, lead L_{II} is showing the maximum deflection say 7 mm. If it is +7 the axis is +60° while if it is –7, the axis is –120°.

DETERMINATION OF QRS AXIS

The QRS axis can be determined by several methods.

Method 1

- Find the lead with smallest or equiphasic deflection.
- Determine the lead at right angles to the first lead.
- See the net deflection in the second lead.
- The axis is directed towards the positive or negative pole of the second lead.

Example A

- Lead with smallest deflection is aVL
- Lead at right angles to aVL is L_{II}
- Major deflection in lead L_{II} is positive

  AXIS is + 60°

Example B

- Lead with smallest deflection is aVR
- Lead at right angles to aVR is L_{III}
- Major deflection in lead L_{III} is negative

  AXIS is –60°

Method 2

- Find the net deflection in leads L_{I} and aVF, which are perpendicular to each other.
- Plot the net deflection in these leads onto their respective axes, on a scale of 0 to 10.
- Drop perpendicular lines from these points and plot a point where these lines intersect.
- Join the centre of the circle to the intersection point and extend it to the circumference.
- The point on the circumference where this line intersects is the QRS axis.

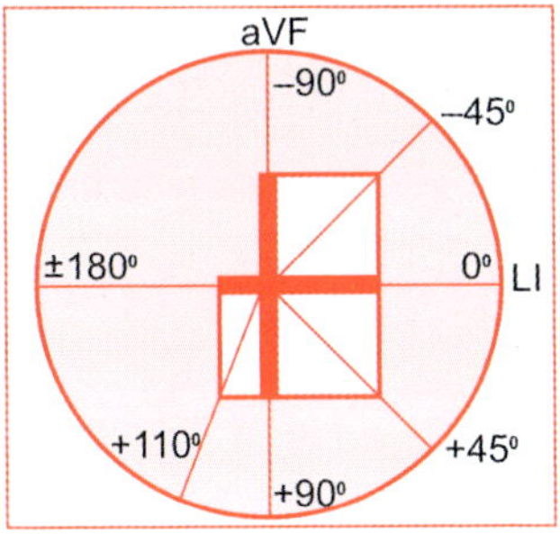

Fig. 4.3: QRS axis determined from leads L_I and aVF

Example A

- Net deflection in L_I is +5
- Net deflection in aVF is 0

AXIS is 0°

Example B

- Net deflection in L_I is +5
- Net deflection in aVF is –5

AXIS is –45° (Fig. 4.3)

Example C

- Net deflection in L_I +6
- Net deflection in aVF + 3

AXIS is + 30°

Method 3

For rapid and easy estimation of QRS axis, just scan the direction of the dominant deflection in leads L_I and aVF whether positive or negative. This gives us the quadrant in which the QRS axis is located (Table 4.1).

Table 4.1: QRS axis quadrant determined from leads L_I and aVF

Main QRS deflection L_I	*aVF*	*QRS axis quadrant*
+ve	+ve	0 to +90°
+ve	–ve	0 to –90°
–ve	+ve	+90 to +180°
–ve	–ve	–90 to –180°

ABNORMALITIES OF QRS AXIS

- Normal QRS axis

  –30° to + 90°

- Right axis deviation

  + 90° to + 180°

  Causes

  Thin built

  Pulmonary disease

  Right ventricular hypertrophy

  Left posterior hemiblock

  Lateral wall infarction

- Left axis deviation

  –30° to –90°

  Causes

  Obesity

  Pregnancy or ascites

  Left ventricular hypertrophy

  Left anterior hemiblock

  Inferior wall infarction

- North-west QRS axis

  –90° to –180°

  Causes

  Congenital heart disease

  Left ventricular aneurysm

  Synonyms

  Indeterminate QRS axis

  Extreme right axis deviation

  NO MAN'S LAND (Fig. 4.4).

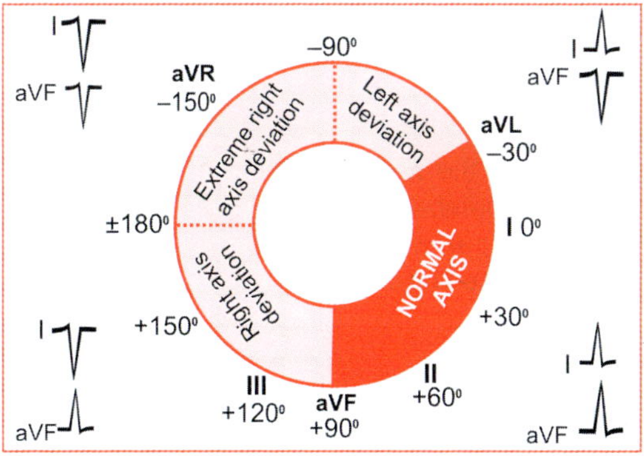

Fig. 4.4: The normal QRS axis and axis deviation

CHAPTER 5

Determination of Heart Rate and Rhythm

THE HEART RATE

The heart rate is simply the number of heart beats per minute. In electrocardiographic terms, the heart rate is the number of cardiac cycles that occur during a 60 second (1 minute) continuous recording of the ECG.

In order to calculate the heart rate from a given ECG strip all that we have to remember is that the ECG paper moves at a speed of 25 mm per second. The rest is all deductive mathematics. Let us see how the heart rate is actually calculated.

Method 1

The ECG paper moves by 25 small squares (each small square = 1/25 = 0.04 seconds), or by 5 large squares (each large square = 5 small squares = 0.04 × 5 = 0.2 seconds) in one second.

If one notes carefully, the vertical line of every fifth large square extends slightly beyond the edge of the graph paper. Therefore, the distance between two such extended lines is one second and the distance between one such line and the sixth line after it is six seconds.

We can count the number of QRS complexes in one such six second interval. Multiplying this number by ten will give us the number of QRS complexes in sixty seconds (one minute), which is the approximate heart rate.

Examples

- There are 8 QRS complexes in a 6 second interval. Heart rate is around 8 × 10 = 80 beats/minute.
- There are 11 QRS complexes in a 6 second interval. Heart rate is around 11 × 10 = 110 beats/minute.

Method 2

The ECG paper moves by 25 small squares in one second. In other words it moves by 25 × 60 = 1500 small squares in 60 seconds or one minute. If the distance between two successive ECG complexes in number of small squares is measured, the number of ECG complexes in one minute will be 1500 divided by that number. This will give us the heart rate in beats per minute (Fig. 5.1).

The interval between two successive P waves (P-P interval) determines the atrial rate and the interval between two successive R waves (R-R interval) determines the ventricular rate. During normal rhythm, the P waves and the QRS complexes track together and therefore, the heart rate calculated by using either the P-P interval or R-R interval will be the same.

To measure the P-P or R-R interval, it is preferable to begin with a P or R wave that is superimposed on a heavy line marking of

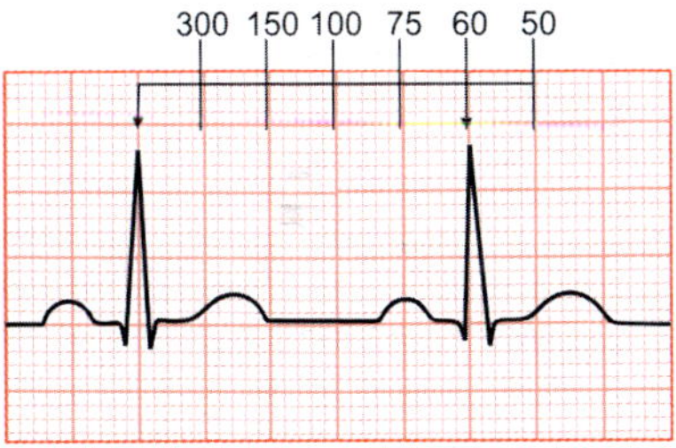

Fig. 5.1: Calculation of heart rate from R-R interval
R-R interval = 25 mm. Heart rate = 60/min

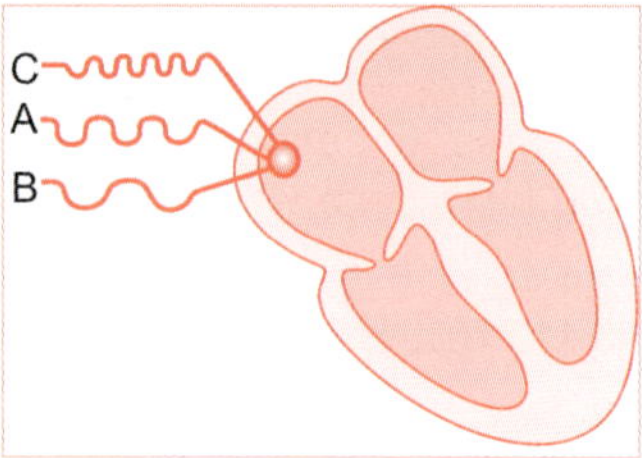

Fig. 5.2: Variation of heart rate
A. Normal rate
B. Bradycardia
C. Tachycardia

a large square. This facilitates the measurement of the interval between it and the next wave, in multiples of 5 mm (one large square = 5 small squares).

A single P-P or R-R interval measurement generally suffices for heart rate determination if the heart beating is regular (equally spaced complexes). If however, the heart beating is irregular (unequally spaced complexes), a mean of 5 or 10 P-P or R-R intervals is taken into account.

Examples

- The R-R interval is 20 mm. Therefore, the heart rate is 1500/ 20- = 75 beats per minute.
- The R-R interval is 12 mm. Therefore, the heart rate is 1500/ 12 = 125 beats per minute.

For rapid heart rate determination, certain standard R-R intervals can be memorized (Table 5.1).

Table 5.1: Determining the heart rate from R-R interval

R-R interval	*Heart rate*
10 mm	1500/10 = 150
12 mm	1500/12 = 125
15 mm	1500/15 = 100
20 mm	1500/20 = 75
25 mm	1500/25 = 60
30 mm	1500/30 = 50

We see that the normal R-R interval ranges from 15 to 25 mm, representing a heart rate of 60 to 100 beats per minute. A short R-R interval (less than 15 mm) denotes tachycardia (heart rate > 100) and a long R-R interval (more than 25 mm) denotes bradycardia (heart rate < 60).

The heart rate range can also be rapidly assessed from the range of R-R interval. For instance:

If the R-R interval is 10 to 15 mm, the heart rate is 100 to 150 per minute.

If the R-R interval is 15 to 20 mm, the heart rate is 75 to 100 per minute.

If the R-R interval is 20 to 25 mm, the heart rate is 60 to 75 per minute.

THE HEART RHYTHM

The rhythm of the heart can be classified on the basis of the following criteria:

- Rate of impulse origin
- Focus of impulse origin
- Pattern of rhythm regularity
- Atrio-ventricular relationship.

Heart Rate

The normal heart rate varies from 60 to 100 beats per minute. A cardiac rhythm at a rate less than 60 beats per minute constitutes bradycardia. A cardiac rhythm at a rate exceeding 100 beats per minute constitutes tachycardia.

We have seen that the P-P interval determines the atrial rate and the R-R interval determines the ventricular rate. Normally, the P-P and R-R intervals are identical and the atrial rate is the same as the ventricular rate. However, under certain circumstances, the atrial and ventricular rates are different and have to be determined separately.

Under normal circumstances when the cardiac rhythm is regular, the measurement of a single R-R interval suffices for heart rate determination as the QRS complexes are equally spaced. If the cardiac rhythm is irregular, that is, the QRS complexes are not equally spaced, a mean of 5 or 10 R-R intervals has to be taken.

On the basis of heart rate, any cardiac rhythm can thus be classified as:

- Normal rate (HR 60-100)
- Bradycardia (HR < 60)
- Tachycardia (HR > 100)

Focus of Origin

The cardiac pacemaker possesses the property of automatic generation of impulses or automaticity. The normal pacemaker is the sinoatrial node (SA node) located in the right atrium.

A cardiac rhythm originating from the SA node is called sinus rhythm. The SA node normally discharges at a rate of 60 to 100 beats per minute. A sinus rhythm at this rate is called normal sinus rhythm.

Besides the SA node, there are other potential pacemakers in the heart such as in the atria, atrioventricular junction and the ventricles. They are known as ectopic or subsidiary pacemakers. The subsidiary pacemakers can discharge at a slower rate than the SA node.

For instance, an atrial or junctional pacemaker can fire 40 to 60 impulses per minute while a ventricular pacemaker can fire 20 to 40 impulses per minute. It is for this reason that the SA node governs the cardiac rhythm by silencing these subsidiary pacemakers. In other words, the subsidiary pacemakers are unable to express their inherent automaticity.

However, under two situations, a subsidiary pacemaker can govern the rhythm of the heart. The first is when impulses generated from the SA node are either insufficient (sinus bradycardia) or they get blocked (SA block) and a subsidiary pacemaker is called upon to take over the cardiac rhythm. The second is when the inherent automaticity of a subsidiary pacemaker is enhanced and it over-rules the SA node to take over the cardiac rhythm.

The former situation, in which a subsidiary pacemaker is called upon to take over the cardiac rhythm, is called an escape rhythm. The subsidiary pacemaker, so to say, escapes the subduing influence of the SA node and expresses its inherent automaticity. The subsidiary pacemaker of an escape rhythm may be junctional or ventricular. Accordingly, an escape rhythm may be classified as:

- Junctional escape rhythm or idiojunctional rhythm
- Ventricular escape rhythm or idioventricular rhythm.

The latter situation, in which a subsidiary pacemaker undergoes enhancement of its inherent automaticity so as to over rule the SA node and take over the cardiac rhythm, is called idiofocal tachycardia. The subsidiary pacemaker of an idiofocal tachycardia may be atrial, junctional or ventricular. Accordingly, an idiofocal tachycardia may be classified as:

- Atrial tachycardia
- Junctional tachycardia
- Ventricular tachycardia.

On the basis of focus of origin, any cardiac rhythm can thus be classified as in Figure 5.3:

- Sinus rhythm
- Atrial rhythm
- Junctional rhythm
- Ventricular rhythm.

Electrocardiographically speaking, the focus of origin of a cardiac rhythm can be reasonably predicted from the morphology of and relationship between P waves and QRS complexes.

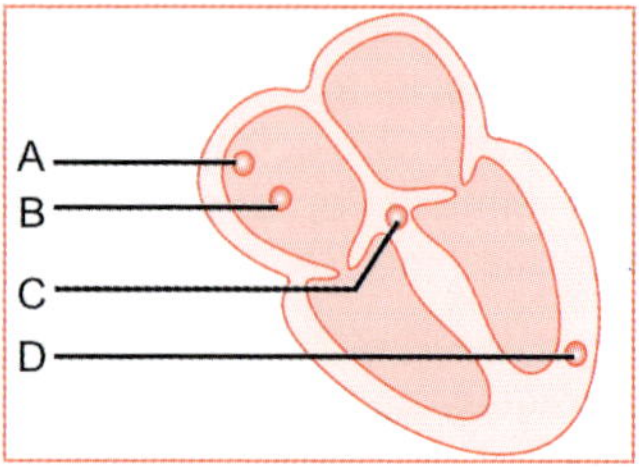

Fig. 5.3: Origin of rhythm
A. Sinus rhythm
B. Atrial rhythm
C. Junctional rhythm
D. Ventricular rhythm

In sinus rhythm, the P waves and QRS complexes are of normal morphology and normally related to each other. In other words, the P wave is upright, the P-R interval is normal and the QRS complex is narrow.

In atrial rhythm, the P wave is different in morphology from the sinus wave and may be inverted due to abnormal sequence of atrial activation. The P-R interval may be short reflecting a shortened atrioventricular conduction time. However, the QRS complex retains its normal narrow configuration as intraventricular conduction of the atrial impulse proceeds as usual.

In junctional rhythm, the P wave is generally inverted and may just precede, just follow or be merged in the QRS complex. This is because the atria are activated retrogradely (from below upwards) from the junctional pacemaker and almost simultaneously with the ventricles. The QRS complexes retain their normal narrow configuration as intraventricular conduction of junctional impulses proceeds as usual.

In ventricular rhythm, either the SA node continues to activate the atria producing upright sinus P waves or the atria are activated by retrograde conduction of ventricular impulses producing inverted P waves. In both cases, the P waves are difficult to discern as the hallmark of a ventricular rhythm is wide QRS complexes in which the P waves are usually buried.

The QRS complex is wide and bizarre in a ventricular rhythm since ventricular activation occurs in a slow, random fashion through the myocardium and not in a rapid, organized fashion through the specialized conduction system (Fig. 5.4).

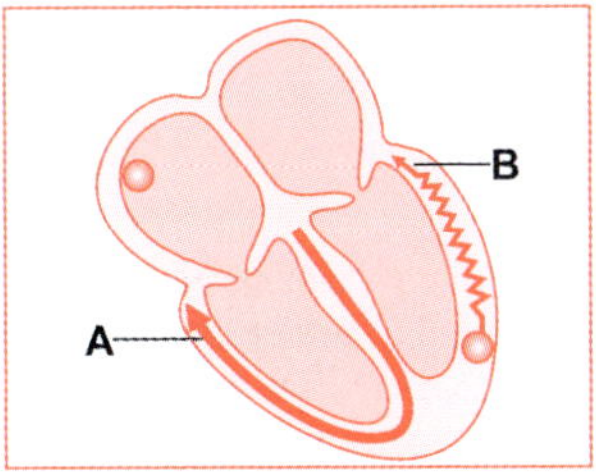

Fig. 5.4: Ventricular activation during any cardiac rhythm
A. Supraventricular rhythm
B. Ventricular rhythm

Pattern of Regularity

The normal cardiac rhythm is regular that is, the interval between the different beats is the same (equally spaced QRS complexes). At times however, the cardiac rhythm may be irregular that is, the QRS complexes are not equally spaced. Irregularity of cardiac rhythm is further of two types, regular irregularity and irregular irregularity.

On the basis of pattern of regularity, any cardiac rhythm can thus be classified as:

- Regular rhythm
- Irregular rhythm
  - regularly irregular rhythm
  - irregularly irregular rhythm

Almost all sinus rhythms including sinus bradycardia and sinus tachycardia as well as fast rhythms such as atrial, junctional and ventricular tachycardias are regular rhythms.

Examples of regularly irregular rhythms are:

- Premature beats during any rhythm
- Regular pauses during any rhythm
- Beats in pairs; bigeminal rhythm.

Fibrillation is the prototype of an irregularly irregular rhythm. Fibrillation is characterized by the functional fragmentation of the atrial or ventricular myocardium into numerous tissue islets

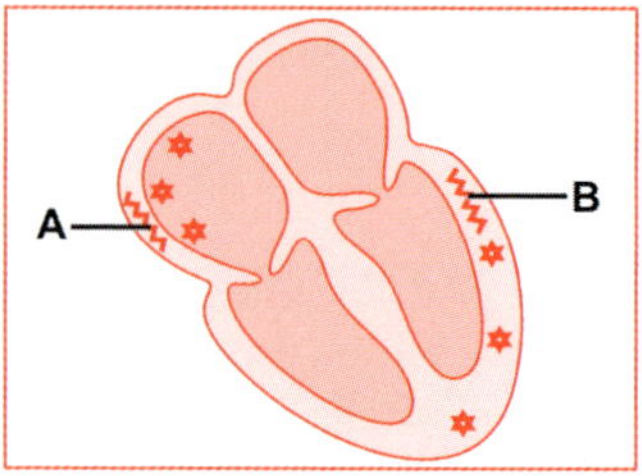

Fig. 5.5: Myocardial activation during fibrillation
A. Atrial fibrillation
B. Ventricular fibrillation

in various stages of excitation and recovery (Fig. 5.5). Myocardial depolarization is thus chaotic and ineffectual in producing haemodynamic pumping.

In atrial fibrillation, the discrete P waves of sinus rhythm are replaced by numerous, small irregularly occurring fibrillatory waves of variable morphology. These fibrillatory waves produce a ragged baseline or a straight line with minimal undulations between QRS complexes.

The R-R interval is highly variable and the heart rate grossly irregular as out of the numerous fibrillatory waves, only a few can activate the ventricles and that too at random. The QRS complexes are normal in morphology as the intraventricular conduction proceeds as usual.

Ventricular fibrillation manifests itself with rapid, irregularly occurring, small deformed deflections, grossly variable in shape, height and width. The regular waveforms of P waves, QRS complexes and T waves are distorted beyond recognition and the baseline seems to waver unevenly.

Atrioventricular Relationship

The normal cardiac activation sequence is such that the electrical impulse from the SA node first activates the atria and then travels downwards through the conducting system to activate the ventricles. We know that atrial depolarization is represented by the P wave and ventricular depolarization is represented by the QRS complex. Therefore, the P wave is followed by the QRS complex and the two are related to each other.

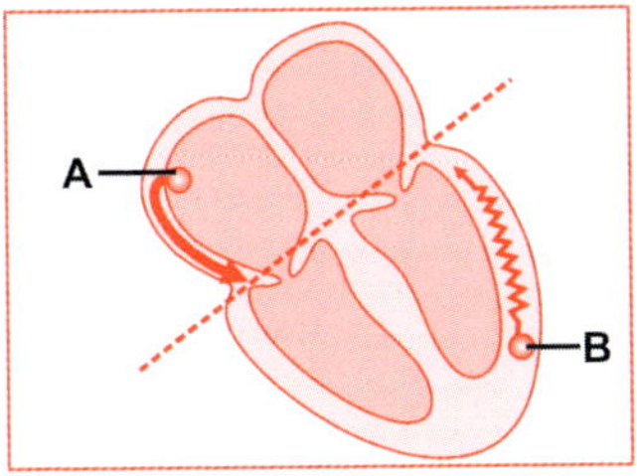

Fig. 5.6: Atrio-ventricular dissociation
A. Atrial rhythm
B. Ventricular rhythm

Imagine, a situation in which the atria are governed by the SA node while the ventricles are governed by a subsidiary pacemaker located in the A-V junction or the ventricle. In that case, the atria and ventricles will beat independent of each other (Fig. 5.6), and the P waves will be unrelated to the QRS complexes. This is precisely what is meant by atrioventricular dissociation (A-V dissociation).

There are various electrocardiographic conditions that produce A-V dissociation. The first situation is one in which a junctional/ventricular pacemaker undergoes an enhancement of automaticity and activates the ventricles at a rate faster than the rate at which the SA node activates the atria.

In that case, the P waves will either be unrelated to the QRS complexes or alternatively, they will be buried in the wide QRS complexes. The R-R intervals may be slightly shorter than the P-P intervals (ventricular rate slightly more than atrial rate). This allows the P-R interval to progressively shorten till the P wave merges into the QRS complex.

Secondly, if there is complete A-V nodal block, no atrial beat is followed by or related to a ventricular beat and the P waves occur independent of the QRS complexes. However, the P-P and R-R intervals are constant. The relative rate of discharge of the atrial and ventricular pacemakers depends upon the condition causing A-V dissociation. This is shown in Table 5.2.

Table 5.2: Different conditions causing A-V dissociation

	Idiojunctional tachycardia	*Idioventricular tachycardia*	*Complete A-V block*
Atrial rate	70-80 (normal)	70-80 (normal)	70-80 (normal)
Junctional rate	70-100 (slightly faster)	—	40-60 (slightly slower) or
Ventricular rate	—	70-100 (slightly faster)	20-40 (much slower)

In A-V dissociation, the P wave retains its normal morphology as the atria are governed by the SA node as usual. The morphology of the QRS complex depends upon the site of the subsidiary pacemaker.

If the pacemaker is junctional, the QRS complex is normal and narrow as ventricular activation occurs through the specialized conduction system. If the pacemaker is ventricular, the QRS complex is abnormal and wide as ventricular activation then occurs through ordinary myocardium.

6

CHAPTER

Abnormalities of the P Wave

NORMAL P WAVE

The P wave is produced by atrial depolarization. It is the sum of right and left atrial activation, the right atrium being activated first since the pacemaker is located in it. The normal P wave meets the following criteria:

- It is upright in most leads (except aVR, V_1)
- It is constant in morphology from beat to beat
- It has a single peak and it is not notched
- It is less than 2.5 mm (0.25 mV) in height
- It is less than 2.5 mm (0.10 sec) in width.

ABSENT P WAVE

The P waves are not discernible in the following conditions:

- *Atrial fibrillation* In atrial fibrillation, P waves are replaced by numerous, small, irregularly occurring fibrillatory waves, producing a ragged base-line.
- *Atrial flutter* In atrial flutter, P waves are replaced by flutter waves (F waves) that give the base-line a corrugated or saw-toothed appearance.
- *Junctional rhythm* In a junctional rhythm, P waves may just precede, just follow or are buried in the QRS complexes due

to near simultaneous activation of the ventricles anterogradely and the atria retrogradely.

- *Ventricular tachycardia* In ventricular tachycardia, P waves are difficult to identify as they lie buried in the wide QRS complexes.
- *Hyperkalemia* In hyperkalemia, P waves are reduced in amplitude or altogether absent. This is associated with tall T waves and wide QRS complexes.

INVERTED P WAVE

The P waves are normally upright in leads L_{II}, L_{III} and aVF, since the atria are activated above downwards towards the inferior leads. If activation of the atria occurs retrogradely from below upwards, the P waves in these leads are negative or inverted. Inverted P waves are thus observed in the following conditions:

- *Junctional rhythm* In a junctional rhythm, inverted P waves may just precede or just follow the QRS complexes.
- *By-pass tract* Inverted P waves are seen if the atria are activated retrogradely through an accessory pathway by-passing the A-V node. This is known as a by-pass tract and occurs in WPW syndrome.

CHANGING P WAVE MORPHOLOGY

Normally, all the P waves in a given ECG strip are of identical morphology, reflecting a constant pattern of atrial activation. If impulses arise from different foci other than the SA node, the pattern of atrial activation varies from beat to beat. This produces P waves of different morphology, known as P' waves. P' waves are observed in the following rhythms:

- *Wandering pacemaker rhythm* In this rhythm the pacemaker, so to say, wanders from one focus to the other. The focus of origin of impulses varies from SA node to atrium to AV junction. This results in P waves of variable morphology.

- *Multifocal atrial tachycardia* In this rhythm, impulses arise from multiple atrial foci to produce an atrial tachycardia or a chaotic pattern of atrial activation. Therefore, the P wave configuration changes from beat to beat.

In both the above rhythms, three kinds of P waves may be observed. Ectopic P' waves are upright but different from sinus P waves and are atrial in origin. Retrograde P' waves are inverted and are junctional in origin. Fusion beats are P waves having a morphology in between that of a sinus P wave and an ectopic P' wave.

TALL P WAVE

The normal P wave is less than 2.5 mm in height. It is the sum of right and left atrial activation, right preceding the left. If the right atrium is enlarged, the deflection of the right atrium is superimposed on the left atrial deflection resulting in a tall P wave exceeding 2.5 mm in height.

Therefore, a tall P wave is representative of right atrial enlargement (Fig. 6.1). A tall P wave is also known as P pulmonale, since it is often caused by pulmonary hypertension or P congenitale, since it may be observed in congenital heart disease.

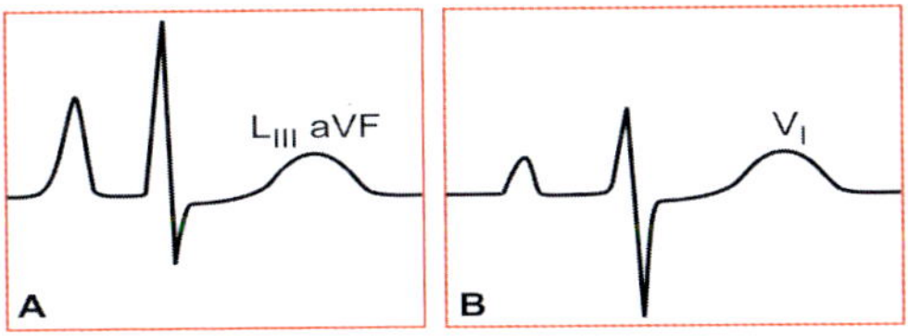

Fig. 6.1: P wave abnormality in right atrial enlargement:
A. Tall, peaked P wave in L_{III}, aVF
B. Initial positive deflection in V_1

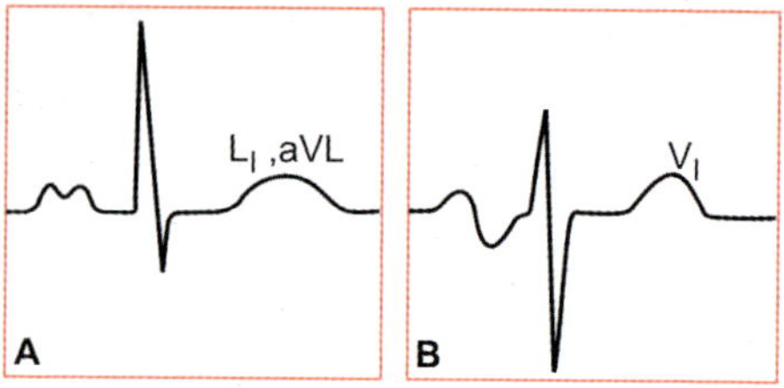

Fig. 6.2: P wave abnormality in left atrial enlargement:
A. Broad, notched P wave in L_I, aVL
B. Terminal negative deflection in V_1

BROAD P WAVE

The normal P wave is less than 2.5 mm or 0.10 sec in width. It is the sum of right and left atrial activation, right preceding the left. If the left atrium is enlarged, the deflection of the left atrium is further delayed after the right atrial deflection, resulting in a broad P wave exceeding 2.5 mm in width. Also, a notch appears on the P wave, between its right and left atrial components.

Therefore, a broad and notched P wave is representative of left atrial enlargement (Fig. 6.2). A broad and notched P wave is also known as P. mitrale since it is often associated with mitral valve disease.

The common causes of atrial enlargement have been enumerated in Table 6.1.

Table 6.1: Various causes of atrial enlargement

	Left atrial enlargement	*Right atrial enlargement*
Intracardiac shunt	Ventricular septal defect	Atrial septal defect
A-V valve disease	Mitral stenosis Mitral regurgitation	Tricuspid stenosis Tricuspid regurgitation
Outflow obstruction	Aortic stenosis	Pulmonary stenosis
Hypertension	Systemic hypertension	Pulmonary hypertension
Myocardial disease	Cardiomyopathy	Corpulmonale

The abnormalities of P wave morphology in right atrial and left atrial enlargement are illustrated in Figure 6.3.

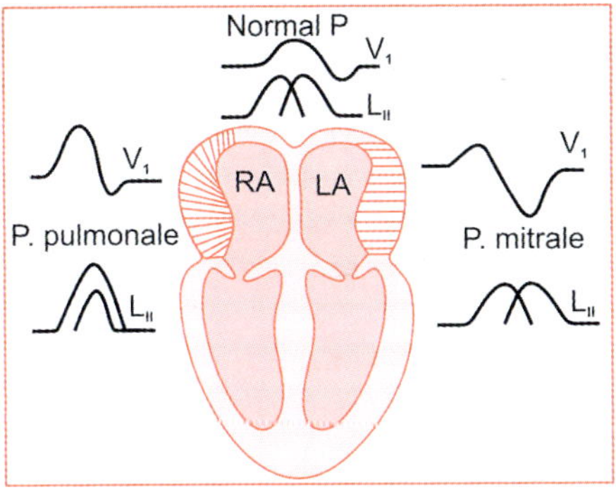

Fig. 6.3: P wave abnormality in right and left atrial enlargement

CHAPTER 7

Abnormalities of the QRS Complex

NORMAL QRS COMPLEX

The QRS complex is produced by ventricular depolarization. It is the sum of synchronized activation of the right and left ventricles. The normal QRS complex meets the following criteria:

- R wave voltage is atleast 5 mm in the limb leads and atleast 10 mm in the precordial leads.
- There is normally no variation in the QRS voltage of consecutive beats in a particular lead.
- The normal QRS axis ranges from –30° to +90° on the hexaxial reference system.
- R wave magnitude increases gradually from lead V_1 to lead V_6 representing transition from right ventricular to left ventricular QRS complexes.
- Physiological q waves are seen in leads L_I, aVL. They are less than 25 percent of the ensuing R wave in size and less than 0.04 second in duration.
- R wave voltage does not exceed 4 mm in lead V_1 and is not more than 25 mm in lead V_5 and V_6.
- The normal S wave is larger than the r wave in lead V_1 and smaller than the R wave in lead V_6. It does not exceed a depth of 7 mm in lead V_6.

- The width of the normal QRS complex does not exceed 0.08 sec or 2 small squares.

LOW-VOLTAGE QRS COMPLEX

The voltage of the R wave in the QRS complex is normally, atleast 5 mm in the limb leads and atleast 10 mm in the precordial leads. If the voltage of the tallest R wave in the limb leads is less than 5 mm and that in the precordial leads is less than 10 mm, the electrocardiogram obtained is called a low voltage graph.

The magnitude of the R wave depends upon the quantum of electrical forces that are generated by the left ventricle as well as on the extent to which these electrical forces are transmitted to the recording electrode.

Therefore, a low voltage graph may be obtained if the myocardium is diseased or if an abnormal substance or tissue intervenes between the epicardial surface of the heart and the recording electrode (Fig. 7.1).

Accordingly, the causes of a low voltage ECG graph can be classified as follows:

- *Due to low voltage generation*

    Hypothyroidism

    Constrictive pericarditis.

    Diffuse myocardial disease

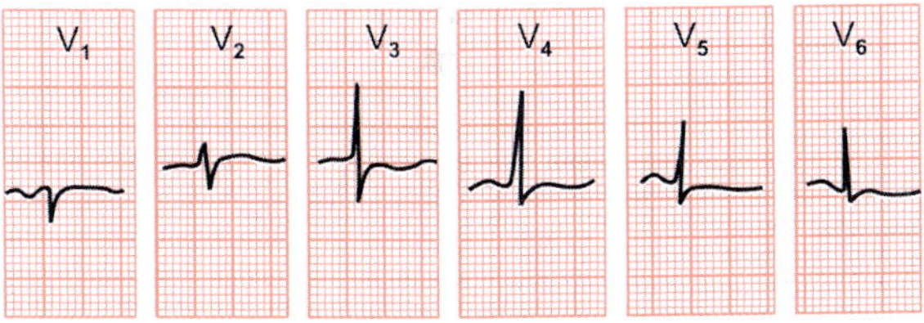

Fig. 7.1: Hypothyroidism: low voltage graph, T wave inversion

- *Due to intervening substance/tissue*

  Adipose tissue in obesity

  Muscle in thick chest wall

  Fluid in pericardial effusion.

  Air in pulmonary emphysema

The cause of a low QRS voltage graph can be assessed by analysis of these parameters:

- The heart rate
- The clinical profile
- The QRS-T shape.

One vital technical point. Before the diagnosis of low QRS voltages is made, it must be ensured that the ECG machine has been properly standardized. Accurate standardization means that a one millivolt current produces a 10 mm tall deflection.

ALTERNATING QRS VOLTAGE

Normally, in a given lead, the voltage of all the QRS complexes is the same. This is because all beats originate from one pacemaker and the voltages have no relation to respiration or any other periodic extracardiac phenomenon.

If the voltage of QRS complexes alternates between high and low in successive beats, the condition is known as electrical alternans (Fig. 7.2). Total electrical alternans refers to a condition wherein, the voltages of P wave, T wave and QRS complex are all variable from beat-to-beat.

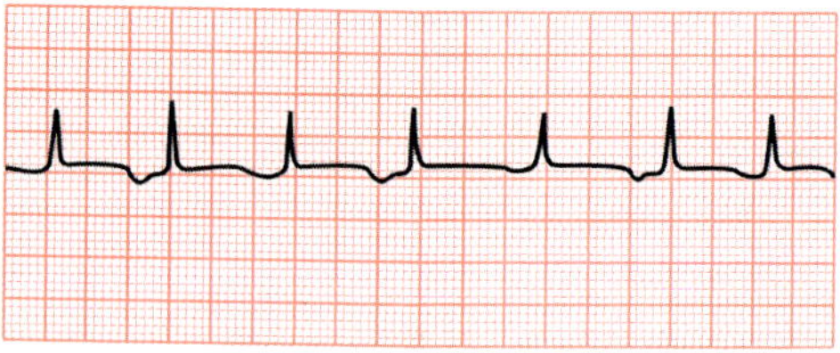

Fig. 7.2: Electrical alternans: varying voltage of QRS complexes

Electrical alternans is caused either by a positional oscillation of the heart within a fluid-filled pericardial sac or a beat-to-beat variation in the aberrancy of intraventricular conduction. Accordingly, the causes of electrical alternans are:

- Moderate to severe pericardial effusion
  - Malignant
  - Tubercular
  - Post-surgical
- Serious organic heart disease
  - Ischemic cardiomyopathy
  - Diffuse myocarditis.

Total electrical alternans is highly suggestive of moderate to severe pericardial effusion with cardiac tamponade or impending tamponade. Electrical alternans of the QRS complex is often clinically associated with cardiomegaly, gallop rhythm and signs of left ventricular decompensation.

ABNORMAL QRS AXIS

The dominant direction of the net electrical forces constitutes the electrical axis of the QRS complex. Normally, these forces are so directed that the QRS axis is in the range of –30° degrees to +90° on the hexaxial reference system.

In other words, the QRS axis falls in the right lower quadrant of the hexaxial system. This means that the main QRS deflection in both leads L_I and aVF is upright. Abnormalities of the QRS axis include:

- Right axis deviation
- Left axis deviation
- Indeterminate axis.

On a scale of 360 degrees (0° to +180° and 0° to –180°), the entire hexaxial system is used to qualify the QRS axis as shown in Table 7.1.

Table 7.1: QRS electrical axis from the hexaxial system	
QRS axis	*Range in degrees*
Normal axis	– 30° to +90°
Left axis deviation	– 30° to –90°
Right axis deviation	+ 90° to +180°
Indeterminate axis	– 90° to –180°

We have seen that although the QRS axis is generally calculated mathematically, we can know the quadrant into which the axis falls by scanning the direction of the main deflection (positive or negative) in leads L_I and aVF. Accordingly, the QRS axis can be classified as in Table 7.2.

Table 7.2: QRS electrical axis from leads L_I and aVF

Main deflection in L_I	*aVF*	*QRS quadrant*	*QRS axis*
+ve	+ve	Right lower	0° to +90°
+ve	–ve	Right upper	0° to –90°
–ve	+ve	Left lower	+90° to +180°
–ve	–ve	Left upper	–90° to –180°

The causes of deviation of the QRS axis are:

- *Right Axis Deviation*
  - Right ventricular hypertrophy
  - Left posterior hemiblock
  - Lateral wall infarction
- *Left Axis Deviation*
  - Obese stocky built
  - Left ventricular hypertrophy

Left anterior hemiblock

Inferior wall infarction.

- *Indeterminate (North-West) Axis*

  Severe right ventricular hypertrophy

  Aneurysm of left ventricular apex.

Deviation of the QRS axis can occur due to various physiological as well as pathological causes. Age and body habitus are important determinants of the QRS axis.

Minor right axis deviation can occur in thin, lean children and adolescents. Minor left axis deviation is normal in obese adults and with abdominal distension due to pregnancy or ascites.

FASCICULAR BLOCK OR HEMIBLOCK

The intraventricular conducting system consists of a bundle of His which divides into right and left bundle branches. The left bundle branch further divides into an anterior fascicle and a posterior fascicle.

A block in conduction down one of the fascicles results in abnormal left ventricular activation known as hemiblock. Thus, we have left anterior hemiblock and left posterior hemiblock. A hemiblock produces significant deviation of the QRS axis.

In left anterior hemiblock, there is qR pattern in lead L_I and rS pattern in lead aVF or left axis deviation (Fig. 7.3A).

In left posterior hemiblock, there is rS pattern in lead L_1 and qR pattern in lead aVF or right axis deviation (Fig. 7.3B).

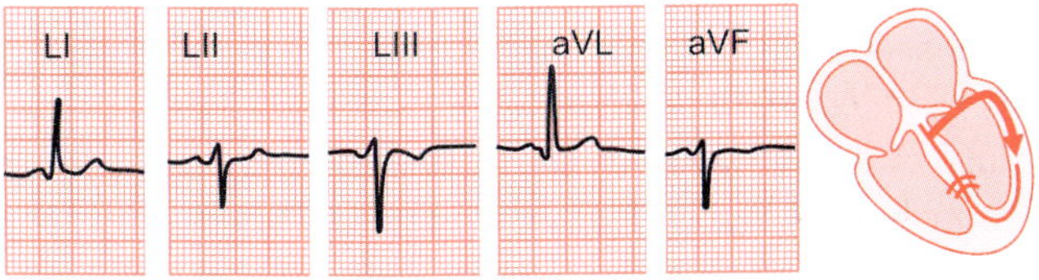

Fig. 7.3A: Left axis deviation due to left anterior fascicular block

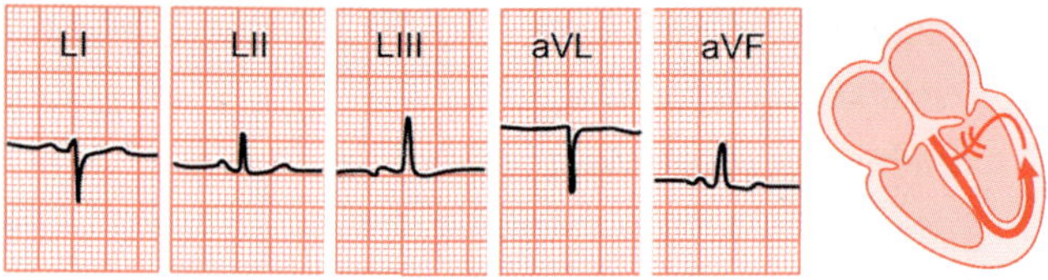

Fig. 7.3B: Right axis deviation due to left posterior fascicular block

Left anterior hemiblock may be observed in:

- Hypertension with LV hypertrophy
- Calcification from aortic valve
- Chronic coronary insufficiency
- Chronic dilated cardiomyopathy
- Fibrocalcerous degeneration.

Left posterior hemiblock rarely occurs in isolated form. It may be observed in:

- Inferior wall infarction
- Right bundle branch block.

NON-PROGRESSION OF R WAVE

Normally, as we move across the precordial leads from lead V_1 to lead V_6, there is a progressive increase in R wave voltage. This is because the right ventricular leads V_1V_2 record rS complexes while the left ventricular leads V_5V_6 record qR complexes.

The change from rS pattern to qR pattern generally occurs in lead V_3 or V_4, which is known as the transition zone.

Failure of the R wave voltage to increase progressively from lead V_1 to lead V_6 is referred to as non-progression of the R wave (Fig. 7.4).

The causes of non-progression of the R wave are:

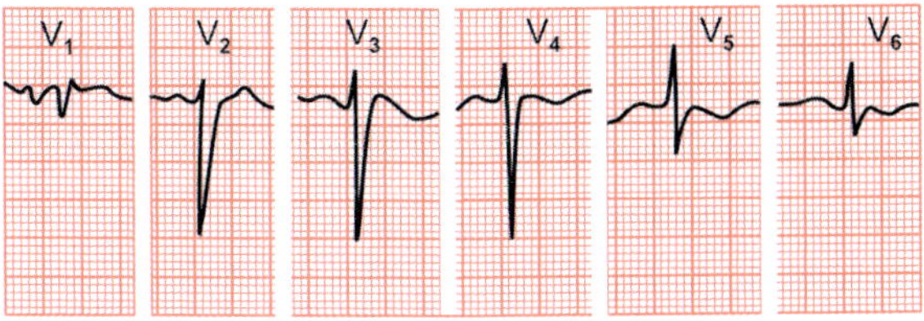

Fig. 7.4: Poor progression of R wave in precordial leads

- Pulmonary emphysema
- Old anterior wall infarction
- Diffuse myocardial disease
- Left ventricular hypertrophy
- Left bundle branch block.

Non-progression of the R wave in precordial leads can occur due to a variety of causes. Knowledge of this fact can avoid the overdiagnosis of ominous conditions like old myocardial infarction.

ABNORMAL Q WAVES

The Q waves are not visible in all ECG leads. Rather, they are normally visible in selected leads where they represent initial septal activation in a direction opposite to activation of the main left ventricular mass.

Physiological Q waves are observed in:

- Leads L_I, aVL, with a horizontal heart position
- Leads L_{III} aVF with a vertical heart position

Criteria for physiological Q waves are:

- They do not exceed 0.04 sec in duration
- They do not exceed 25 percent of R wave.

Pathological Q waves are most commonly due to necrosis of heart muscle or myocardial infarction. This is a result of occlusion

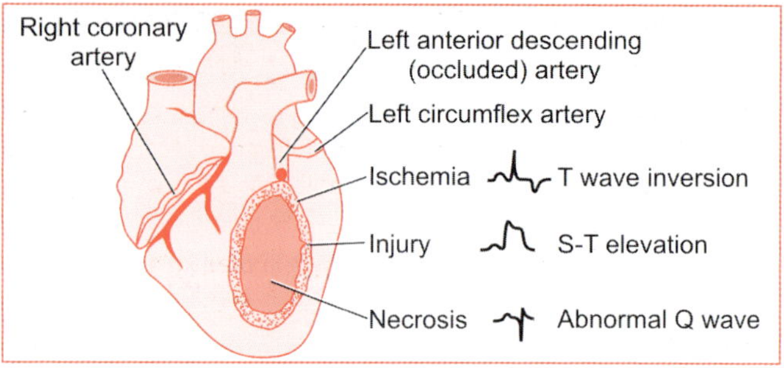

Fig. 7.5: Zones of myocardial infarction and their ECG features

of a coronary artery by a thrombus (Fig. 7.5). Why pathological Q waves appear in myocardial infarction needs to be understood. Infarcted (necrosed) myocardial tissue is electrically inert and does not get depolarized. If an electrode is placed over this "electrical hole", it records activation of the opposite ventricular wall from the endocardial to epicardial surface.

Since, this direction of activation is away from the electrode, the recorded deflection is negative and is called the Q wave (Fig. 7.6). The Q wave may be followed by a small r wave or there may be an entirely negative deflection called the QS complex.

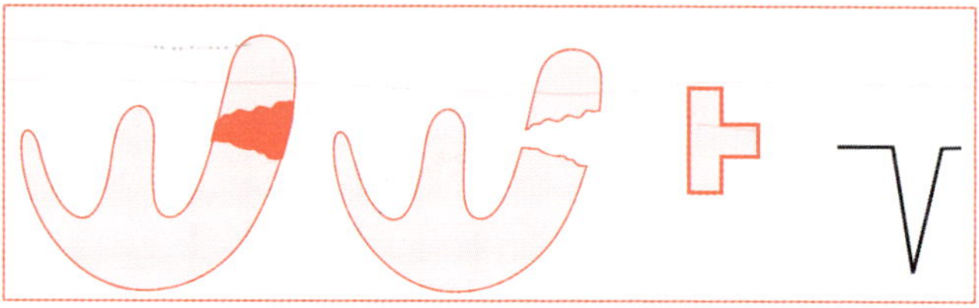

Fig. 7.6: An electrode placed over a transmural infarct records a negative deflection. The "electrical hole" effect

Pathological Q waves meet the following criteria:

- more than or equal to 0.04 sec in duration
- more than 25 percent of R wave in size

- present in leads besides those with normal q waves
- present in several leads and not an isolated lead.

Pathological Q waves occur commonly but not always due to myocardial infarction. Severe reversible myocardial ischemia as in severe angina, hypoxia, hypothermia or hypoglycemia may cause transient appearance of Q waves.

Absence of Q waves does not rule out the possibility of myocardial infarction. Q waves may be absent in the following types of infarction: small infarction, right ventricular infarction, posterior wall infarction, atrial infarction and fresh infarction with delayed ECG changes.

The location of Q waves can help to localize the area of infarction as tabulated below in Table 7.3.

Table 7.3: Area of infarction determined from Q wave location

Location of Q wave	*Area of infarction*
V_1V_2	Septal
V_3V_4	Anterior
$V_5V_6L_IaVL$	Lateral
V_{1-4}	Anteroseptal
$V_{3-6}L_IaVL$	Anterolateral
$V_{1-6}L_IaVL$	Extensive anterior
L_IaVL	High lateral
$L_{II}L_{III}aVF$	Inferior

ABNORMALLY TALL R WAVES

The r wave voltage in lead V_1 represents rightward forces while the R wave height in lead V_6 represents left ventricular forces. Normally, the R wave amplitude does not exceed 4 mm in lead V_1 and does not exceed 25 mm in lead V_6. Also, the R wave height is less than S wave depth (R/S ratio less than 1) in lead

V_1 and more than the S wave depth (R/S ratio more than 1) in lead V_6.

A R wave greater than 4 mm in lead V_1 is considered tall. Causes of tall R waves in lead V_1 are:

- Right ventricular hypertrophy
- Right bundle branch block
- Right ventricular dominance
- Posterior wall infarction
- Mirror-image dextrocardia
- The WPW syndrome.

A R wave greater than 25 mm in lead V_6 is considered tall. Causes of tall R waves in lead V_6 are:

- Left ventricular hypertrophy
- Left bundle branch block.

Right Ventricular Hypertrophy (RVH)

The tall R wave in lead V_1 due to right ventricular hypertrophy reflects the increased electrical forces generated by the hypertrophied right ventricular myocardium.

The voltage criteria of RVH are:

- R wave in V_1 more than 4 mm
- R/S ratio in V_1 more than 1
- S wave in V_6 more than 7 mm
- R in V_1 + S in V_6 more than 10 mm.

Besides voltage criteria, other features of RVH are:

- Right axis deviation of the QRS complex
- S-T segment depression and T wave inversion in leads V_1 and V_2: the RV strain pattern (Fig. 7.7)
- Right atrial enlargement: P. pulmonale.

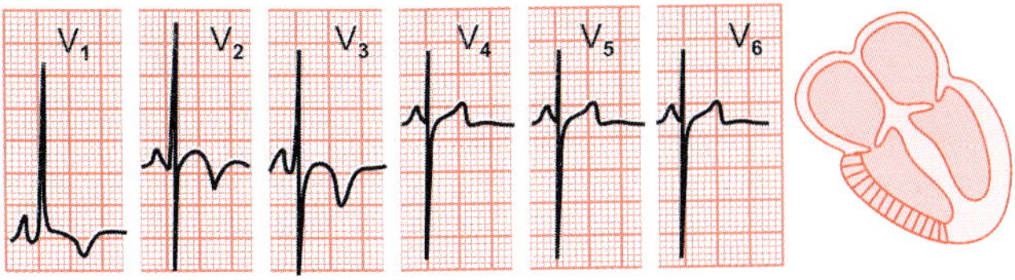

Fig. 7.7: Right ventricular hypertrophy:
tall R wave in V_1 to V_3
rS pattern in V_4 to V_6

The causes of RVH can be classified into causes of pulmonary hypertension and those of pulmonary stenosis. These are:

- *Pulmonary Hypertension*

  Congenital heart disease (intracardiac shunt)

  Mitral valve disease (stenosis or regurgitation)

  Chronic pulmonary disease (corpulmonale)

  Primary pulmonary hypertension (idiopathic).

- *Pulmonary Stenosis (PS)*

  Isolated congenital PS

  PS of Fallot's tetralogy.

In pulmonary hypertension, there is increased resistance to blood flow in the pulmonary vasculature. In pulmonary stenosis, there is obstruction to right ventricular outflow at the level of pulmonary valve.

Right ventricular hypertrophy is a common but by no means, the only cause of tall R waves in lead V_1. It needs to be differentiated from the following conditions that also produce tall R waves in lead V_1.

Persistent Juvenile Pattern

The right ventricle is the dominant ventricle in childhood. Sometimes, the juvenile pattern of right ventricular dominance persists into adulthood to cause a dominantly upright deflection in lead V_1.

Right Bundle Branch Block (RBBB)

In RBBB, the dominant deflection in lead V_1 is upright. But close analysis of the QRS complex reveals a wide deflection (>0.12 sec in width) with a triphasic contour that produces a M-pattern or RsR' configuration.

Posterior Wall Infarction

None of the electrocardiographic leads is oriented towards the posterior wall of the heart. Therefore, the diagnosis of posterior wall infarction is made from the inverse of classical changes of infarction in lead V_1.

These include a tall R wave and an upright T wave which are the reverse of a deep Q wave and an inverted T wave. Note that posterior wall infarction is the only cause of tall R wave in V_1 in which the T wave is also tall and upright.

Mirror-image Dextrocardia

In mirror-image dextrocardia, since the heart lies in the right side of the chest and lead V_1 overlies the left ventricle, the R wave is tallest in lead V_1 and diminishes towards lead V_6.

The WPW Syndrome

The WPW syndrome or pre-excitation syndrome is often associated with upright QRS complexes in right precordial leads V_1, V_2. Other electrocardiographic features of WPW syndrome include a short P-R interval and a delta wave deforming the normally smooth ascending limb of the R wave.

Left Ventricular Hypertrophy (LVH)

The tall R wave in lead V_5, V_6 due to left ventricular hypertrophy reflects the increased electrical forces generated by the hypertrophied left ventricular myocardium.

The voltage criteria of LVH are:

- R wave in V_5/V_6 more than 27 mm
- R wave in aVL more than 11 mm
- S in V_1 + R in V_5/V_6 more than 37 mm
- R in L_I + S in L_{III} more than 25 mm
- Tallest R + deepest S more than 45 mm

Besides voltage criteria, other features of LVH are:

- Left axis deviation of the QRS complex.
- S-T segment depression and T wave inversion in leads V_5 and V_6: LV strain pattern (Fig. 7.8).
- Left atrial enlargement: P mitrale.

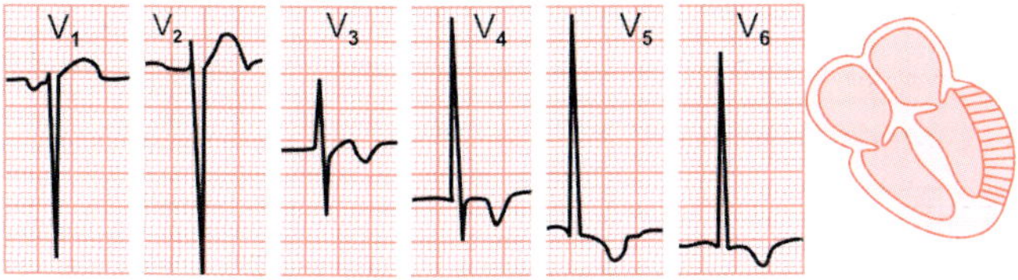

Fig. 7.8: Left ventricular hypertrophy: tall R wave in V_5, V_6 deep S wave in V_1, V_2

The causes of LVH can be classified into causes of systolic LV overload and those of diastolic LV overload. These are:

- *Systolic LV Overload*
  - Systemic hypertension
  - Aortic stenosis
    - Valvular
    - Subvalvular
  - Coarctation of aorta
- *Diastolic LV Overload*
  - Aortic regurgitation
  - Mitral incompetence
  - Intracardiac shunt
    - Ventricular septal defect
    - Patent ductus arteriosus.

In systolic overload, there is increased resistance to outflow of arterial blood from the left ventricle. In diastolic overload, there is an increased inflow of venous blood to the left ventricle.

Left ventricular hypertrophy is a common but by no means, the only cause of tall R wave in V_6. It needs to be differentiated from the following conditions that also cause tall R wave in lead V_6.

- *Voltage criteria alone* The voltage criteria of LVH can be fulfilled by high cardiac output states such as anaemia, thyrotoxicosis and beri-beri. Similarly, strenuous exercisers, athletes and marathon runners, can have tall R waves in lead V_6.

  However, in these conditions, the voltage criteria are not accompanied by other ECG features of LVH such as left axis deviation, strain pattern or P. mitrale. Moreover, their clinical evaluation is unremarkable. Therefore, one must be careful before diagnosing left ventricular hypertrophy by voltage criteria alone.

- *Left bundle branch block (LBBB)* In LBBB, the QRS deflection in lead V_6 is tall. But close analysis of the QRS complex reveals a wide deflection (> 0.12 sec in width) with a triphasic contour that produces a M-pattern or RsR' configuration.
- *Left ventricular diastolic overload* In true left ventricular hypertrophy or systolic overload, the tall R wave without a preceding Q wave is classically associated with depression of the S-T segment and inversion of the T wave, the so called left ventricular strain pattern.

  Left ventricular diastolic overload can be differentiated from systolic overload by certain subtle differences. In diastolic overload, the tall R wave is preceded by a deep narrow Q wave and associated with a tall and upright T wave.

ABNORMALLY DEEP S WAVES

The S wave in lead V_1 represents left ventricular activation while in lead V_6 it represents right ventricular activation. Normally, the S wave depth in lead V_1 is greater than the r wave height. Also, the s wave is much smaller than the R wave in lead V_6 and does not exceed 7 mm in depth.

In lead V_1, if the s wave is smaller than the R wave and the R/S ratio is greater than 1, it indicates right ventricular dominance or hypertrophy (Fig. 7.7). If the sum of S wave voltage in lead V_1 and R wave voltage in lead V_6 exceeds 37 mm, it indicates left ventricular hypertrophy (Fig. 7.8).

In lead V_6, if the S wave is greater than the R wave, it indicates right ventricular dominance or non-progression of R wave in precordial leads. S wave voltage greater than 7 mm in lead V_6 indicates right ventricular hypertrophy.

ABNORMALLY WIDE QRS COMPLEXES

The QRS complex represents depolarization of the entire ventricular myocardium. Since the right and left ventricles are depolarized in a synchronous fashion, the normal QRS width does not exceed 0.04 to 0.08 sec (1 to 2 small squares) on the horizontal or time axis.

If the QRS complex is wider than 0.08 sec, it means that either the two ventricles are activated asynchronously or ventricular conduction is slow. Causes of wide QRS complexes are:

- Bundle branch block
  - Right bundle branch block
  - Left bundle branch block
- *Intraventricular conduction defect*
  - Antiarrhythmic drugs, e.g. quinidine
  - Electrolyte imbalance, e.g. hyperkalemia
  - Myocardial disease, e.g. cardiomyopathy
- *Ventricular pre-excitation*
  - WPW syndrome
  - LGL syndrome
- *Wide QRS arrhythmias*
  - Supraventricular arrhythmias with aberrant ventricular conduction
  - Ventricular arrhythmias.

The causes of wide QRS complexes can also be classified according to the width of the complexes:

- *QRS Width 0.09-0.10 sec*

  Left anterior or posterior hemiblock

  Partial intraventricular conduction defect

- *QRS Width 0.11-0.12 sec*

  Incomplete bundle branch block

  Intraventricular conduction defect

  Ventricular pre-excitation syndrome

- *QRS Width > 0.12 sec*

  Bundle branch block

  Wide QRS arrhythmias.

Bundle Branch Block

Bundle branch block denotes a delay or block of conduction in one of the branches of the bundle of His. Accordingly, we can have right bundle branch block (RBBB) and left bundle branch block (LBBB). Bundle branch block produces widening of the QRS complex because of delayed activation of one of the ventricles, right ventricle in RBBB and left ventricle in LBBB, which occurs slowly through ordinary myocardium and not through the specialized conduction system.

An incomplete bundle branch block results in a QRS width of 0.11 to 0.12 sec while in a complete block the QRS width exceeds 0.12 sec. Bundle branch block produces a RSR' pattern or M-shaped QRS deflection.

In RBBB, the RSR' pattern is observed in lead V_1, the R' wave representing delayed right ventricular activation (Fig. 7.9A). In LBBB, the M-shaped pattern is observed in lead V_6, the notched R wave representing delayed left ventricular activation (Fig. 7.9B). The RSR' complex is followed by S-T segment depression and T wave inversion which together constitute secondary ST-T changes of bundle branch block.

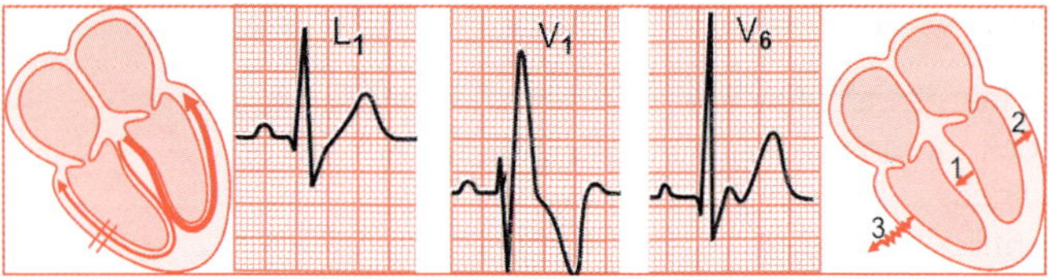

Fig. 7.9A: Right bundle branch block:
M-shaped complex in V_1
deep slurred S wave in L_I, V_6

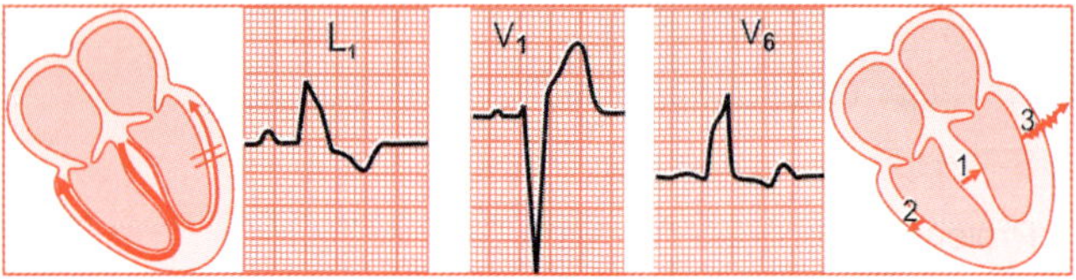

Fig. 7.9B: Left bundle branch block:
M-shaped complex in L_I, V_6
wide QS complex in V_1

Bundle branch block often indicates organic heart disease, more so LBBB, since RBBB is occasionally observed in normal individuals. Causes of bundle branch block are:

- Myocardial infarction (recent or old)
- Systemic hypertension (long-standing)
- Aortic valve disease (calcific stenosis)
- Cardiomyopathy (or myocarditis)
- Fibrocalcerous disease (degenerative)
- Cardiac trauma (accidental or surgical).

Intraventricular Conduction Defect

An intraventricular conduction defect (IVCD) refers to a delay or block in conduction in the Purkinje system, distal to the bundle branches. It produces widening of the QRS complex since the ventricular muscle has to be activated through ordinary myocardium instead of the specialized conduction tissue. As we have seen earlier, an IVCD may occur due to anti-arrhythmic drugs, electrolyte imbalance or primary myocardial disease.

Antiarrhythmic drugs such as quinidine, widen the QRS complex. A widening beyond 25 percent of the base-line value is an indication of drug toxicity. Other ECG effects of quinidine and similar drugs are:

- S-T depression and T inversion
- Prolongation of Q-T interval.
- Prominence of U wave (Fig. 7.10)
- Ventricular arrhythmias.

Hyperkalemia (serum K^+ more than 9 mEq/L) results in a QRS complex that is wide and bizarre. Other ECG features of hyperkalemia are:

- Tall peaked T waves (Fig. 7.11)
- Short Q-T interval
- Absent P waves
- A-V block or ventricular arrhythmias.

Disease processes primarily affecting the myocardium such as cardiomyopathy or myocarditis produce total distortion and widening of the QRS complex. Low voltages of these complexes may cause poor progression of R wave in precordial leads.

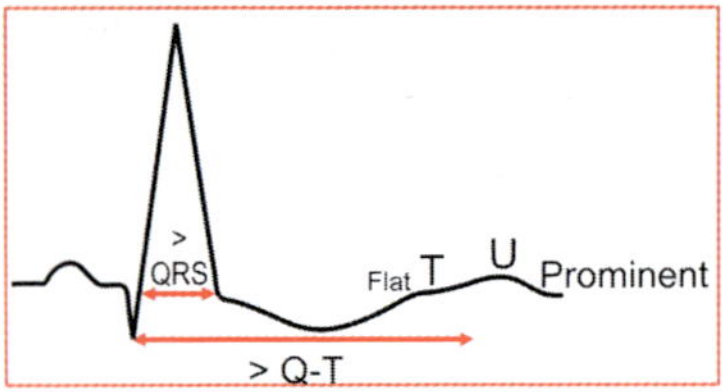

Fig. 7.10: Effects of quinidine on the P-QRS-T

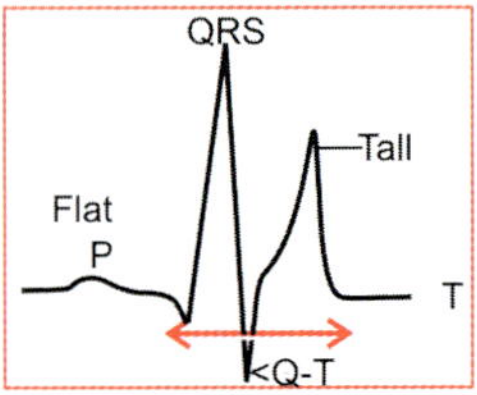

Fig. 7.11: Effects of hyperkalemia on the P-QRS-T

Ventricular Pre-excitation (WPW Syndrome)

The WPW syndrome is an entity in which an accessory pathway or by-pass tract called the bundle of Kent connects the atrial to the ventricular myocardium, without passing through the A-V node.

Conduction of impulses down this tract results in premature ventricular activation, also called pre-excitation, since the A-V nodal delay is by-passed. Conduction of an impulse through the usual conduction system follows the pre-excitation. The WPW syndrome is associated with the following ECG features:

- *Wide QRS complex* The QRS complex is wide since it is the sum of ventricular pre-excitation and normal ventricular activation.

- *Delta wave* Pre-excitation of the ventricle produces a slur on the ascending limb of R wave, the delta wave.
- *Short P-R interval* The P-R interval is short because ventricular depolarization begins early after the P wave, having by-passed the A-V nodal delay.
- *ST-T changes* S-T segment depression and T wave inversion are secondary to the abnormality of the QRS complex (Fig. 7.12).

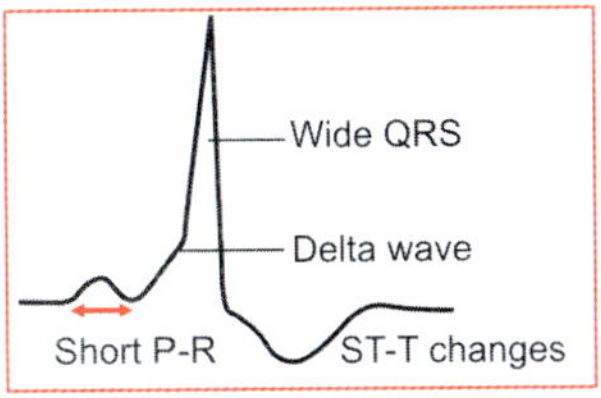

Fig. 7.12: Abnormal P-QRS-T in WPW syndrome

The clinical significance of WPW syndrome lies in the fact that it predisposes an individual to arrhythmias particularly paroxysmal atrial tachycardia, atrial fibrillation and even ventricular tachycardia or ventricular fibrillation.

8

CHAPTER

Abnormalities of the T Wave

NORMAL T WAVE

The T wave is produced by ventricular repolarization and follows the QRS complex. The normal T wave fulfills the following criteria:

- It is upright in most leads (except aVR, L_{III}, V_1)
- It is taller in lead V_6 than in lead V_1 and taller in L_I than in lead L_{III}
- It does not exceed 5 mm in height in limb leads and 10 mm in precordial leads.

INVERTED T WAVE

The T wave is considered to be the most unstable component of the ECG graph. Therefore, change in polarity of the T wave or T wave inversion is one of the most common ECG abnormalities.

The significance of flattening or reduction in height of the T wave is similar to that of T wave inversion. Since inversion of the T wave is often associated with depression of the S-T segment, together they are referred to as ST-T changes.

As the T wave is an unstable deflection, it is not surprising that T wave inversion can be caused by a wide variety of aetiological factors. The causes of T wave inversion can be classified as follows:

NON-SPECIFIC CAUSES

- *Physiological states*

  Heavy meals

  Smoking

  Anxiety

  Tachycardia

  Hyperventilation

- *Extra-cardiac disorders*

  Systemic, e.g. haemorrhage, shock

  Cerebral, e.g. vascular accident

  Abdominal, e.g. pancreatitis, cholecystitis

  Respiratory, e.g. pulmonary embolism

  Endocrine, e.g. hypothyroidism.

SPECIFIC CAUSES

- *Primary abnormality*

  Pharmacological, e.g. digitalis, quinidine

  Metabolic, e.g. hypokalemia, hypothermia

  Myocardial, e.g. cardiomyopathy, myocarditis

  Pericardial, e.g. pericarditis, pericardial effusion

  Ischemic, e.g. coronary insufficiency, infarction

- *Secondary abnormality*

  Ventricular hypertrophy

  Bundle branch block

  WPW syndrome.

T wave inversion lacks specificity as a diagnostic indicator. Since inversion of the T wave can be caused by certain physiological states and non-cardiac diseases, it highlights the importance of viewing T inversion in the light of clinical data.

One should be careful before diagnosing myocardial ischemia only by ECG criteria. T wave inversion should be interpreted carefully in the presence of upper abdominal and respiratory diseases, when the clinical picture may be confused with that of heart disease. Similarly, any survivor of a cerebrovascular accident should not be presumed to have coronary artery disease if the ECG shows T wave inversion.

Cardiovascular drugs like digitalis and quinidine can cause T wave inversion and S-T segment depression. With digitalis therapy, the S-T segment and T wave resemble the mirror-image of the correction mark sign (√) (Fig. 8.1A).

When these changes are confined to leads V_5, V_6, they indicate digitalis administration. Changes occurring in most leads are suggestive of digitalis intoxication.

Quinidine also causes T wave inversion and S-T segment depression but unlike digitalis, quinidine also widens the QRS complex and prolongs the Q-T interval (Fig. 8.1B).

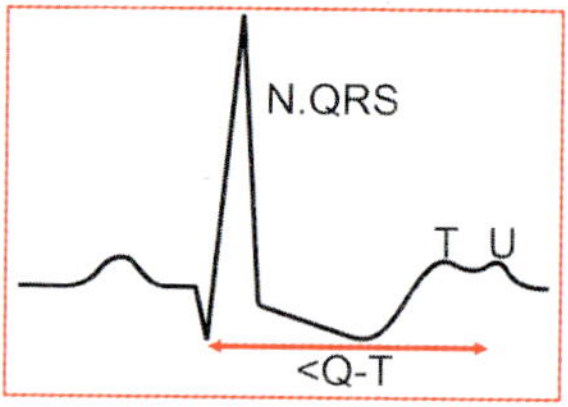

Fig. 8.1A: Effects of digitalis on the P-QRS-T

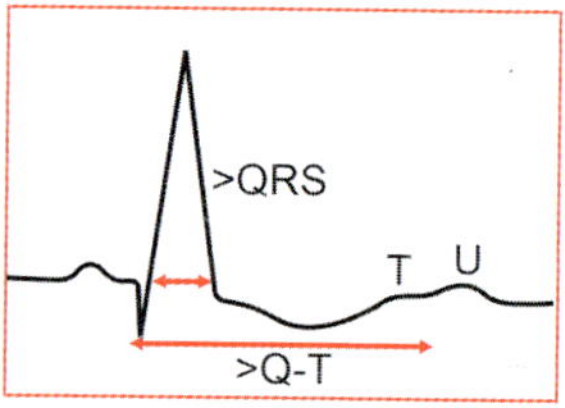

Fig. 8.1B: Effects of quinidine on the P-QRS-T

Hypokalemia is an important cause of T wave change. The T wave is either reduced in amplitude, flattened or inverted. This is associated with prominence of the U wave that follows the T wave. A low T wave followed by a prominent U wave produces a 'camel-hump' effect while a flat T with a prominent U falsely suggests prolongation of the Q-T interval (Fig. 8.2).

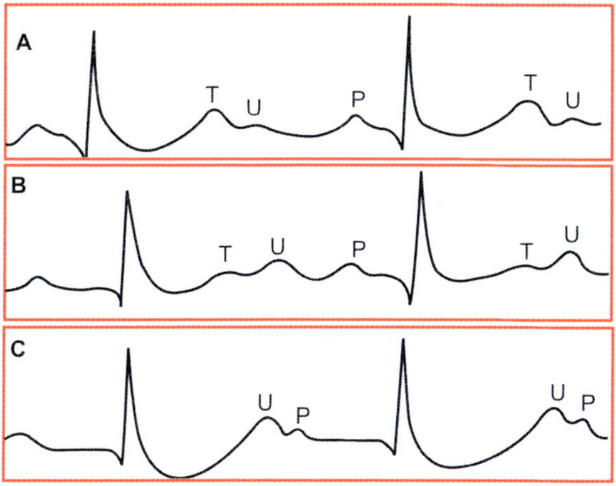

Fig. 8.2: Effects of progressively increasing hypokalemia

Causes of hypokalemia include dietary deficiency of potassium, gastrointestinal losses in the form of vomiting and diarrhoea as well as diuretic and steroid therapy. The importance of hypokalemia in cardiac patients on diuretic treatment lies in the fact that hypokalemia aggravates digitalis toxicity and likelihood of ventricular arrhythmias.

Clinical features of hypokalemia are fatigue, leg cramps and neuromuscular paralysis. Treatment of hypokalemia is potassium administration, either dietary or pharmacological and correction of the underlying cause.

Primary diseases of the myocardium such as cardiomyopathy and acute myocarditis produce T wave inversion and S-T segment depression. These changes are often associated with wide QRS complexes due to intraventricular conduction defect.

During the acute stage of pericarditis, the S-T segment is elevated and the T wave is upright. Once the S-T segment has returned to the baseline, the T wave undergoes inversion that may persist for a long time.

In pericardial effusion, T wave inversion is associated with low voltage QRS complexes. A similar pattern is observed in hypothyroidism (myxoedema) with the difference that while pericardial effusion causes tachycardia, hypothyroidism is accompanied by bradycardia.

Clinically speaking, coronary artery disease with myocardial ischemia or infarction is the most important cause of T wave inversion. Acute coronary insufficiency produces coving (convexity) of the S-T segment and T wave inversion (Fig. 8.3). In non-Q myocardial infarction, a similar pattern is observed.

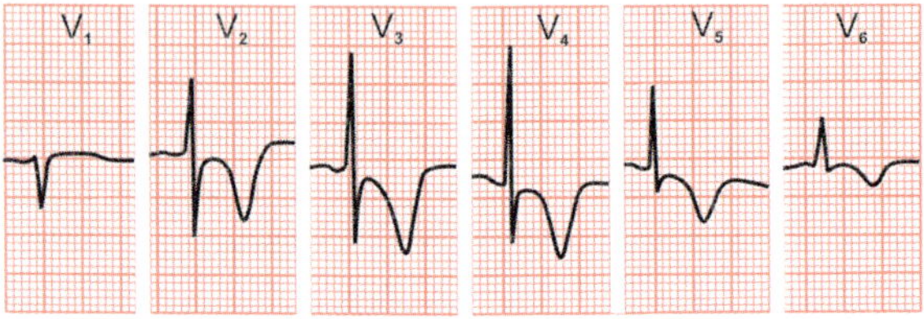

Fig. 8.3: Acute non-Q wave anterior wall myocardial infarction: convex S-T segment; symmetrical, inverted T wave

The two conditions can be differentiated by the fact that in acute coronary insufficiency, the chest pain is of short duration, cardiac enzyme titres (CPK, SGOT) are normal and the ECG changes rapidly revert to normal with treatment. In non-Q myocardial infarction, there is history of prolonged chest pain, blood levels of cardiac enzymes are raised and the ECG changes persist for a longer period.

In the fully evolved phase of Q-wave myocardial infarction, T wave inversion is associated with elevation (convex upwards) of the S-T segment (Fig. 8.4). This is in contrast to the T wave inversion observed in pericarditis which occurs after the elevated (concave upwards) S-T segment has nearly returned to the baseline.

The inverted T wave of ischemic heart disease (coronary insufficiency or myocardial infarction) has certain characteristic

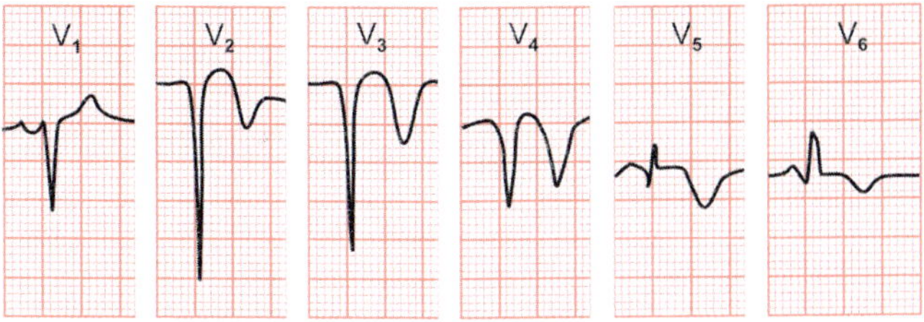

Fig. 8.4: Acute extensive anterior wall myocardial infarction fully evolved phase: QS in V_1 to V_4, qR in V_5 to V_6

features. The T wave is symmetrical, the apex is midway between its two limbs and peaked like an arrow-head (Fig. 8.3).

A subtle evidence of myocardial ischemia is that the T wave amplitude in lead L_I is less than in L_{III} and that in lead V_6 is less than in V_1 (Fig. 8.5).

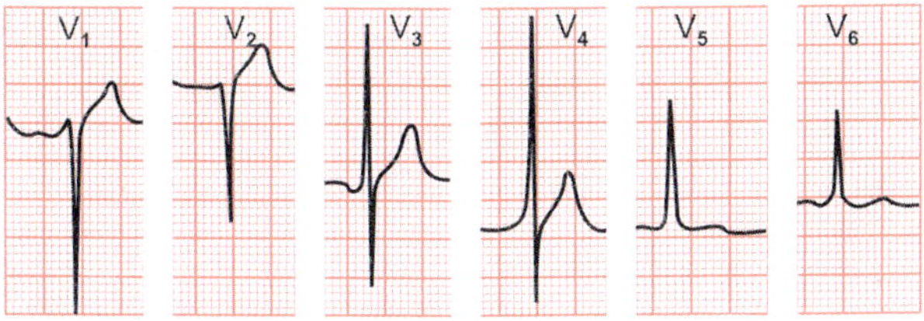

Fig. 8.5: Coronary insufficiency: T wave in V_1 is taller than in V_6

Conditions associated with abnormal QRS morphology may also cause T wave inversion in the leads where the QRS complexes are upright. Three classical examples are ventricular hypertrophy, bundle branch block and WPW syndrome.

The T wave inversion in these conditions is secondary to abnormal ventricular depolarization or intraventricular conduction and is called secondary T wave inversion.

The characteristic feature of secondary T wave inversion is that it is asymmetrical, with the distal limb steeper than the proximal limb and the apex is blunt (Fig. 8.6).

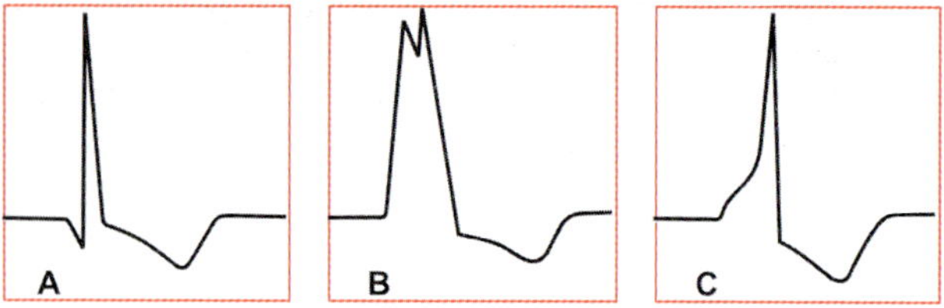

Fig. 8.6: Causes of secondary T wave inversion
A. Ventricular hypertrophy
B. Bundle branch block
C. WPW syndrome

T wave inversion secondary to ventricular hypertrophy occurs in leads showing tall R waves. This along with S-T segment depression constitutes the pattern of systolic overload or ventricular strain (Fig. 8.7). It is secondary to increased myocardial tension or relative ischemia of the hypertrophied myocardium.

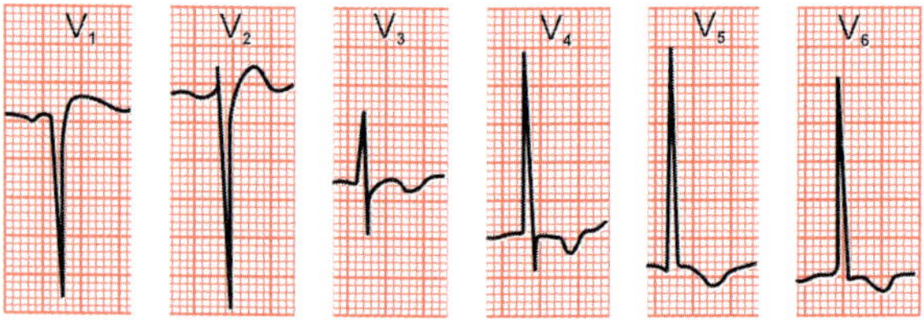

Fig. 8.7: Left ventricular hypertrophy with ventricular strain: depressed S-T segment; inverted T wave in V_4 to V_6

In bundle branch block, the T wave is generally opposite to the direction of the QRS deflection and constitutes secondary T wave inversion. If the T wave is upright in leads showing a positive QRS deflection, associated myocardial ischemia should be considered.

In WPW syndrome, the T wave is inverted in leads showing a wide and upright deflection. It reflects abnormal repolarization secondary to pre-excitation of the ventricle.

T wave inversion in nearly all ECG leads is generally due to non-specific causes, a metabolic abnormality or a diffuse process affecting the myocardium or pericardium. Regional inversion of the T wave in specific leads can be caused by specific aetiological factors such as:

- *In Leads L_I, aVL, V_5, V_6*
  - Lateral wall ischemia/infarction
  - Left ventricular hypertrophy
  - Left bundle branch block
  - Digitalis effect or toxicity
- *In Leads V_1, V_2, V_3*
  - Anteroseptal ischemia/infarction
  - Right ventricular hypertrophy
  - Right bundle branch block
  - WPW syndrome, Type A
- *In Leads L_{II}, L_{III}, aVF*
  - Inferior wall ischemia/infarction
  - Mitral valve prolapse syndrome

TALL T WAVE

The T wave exceeding a voltage of 5 mm in the standard leads and 10 mm in precordial leads is considered tall.

The causes of tall T waves are:

- Hyperkalemia (Fig. 8.8)
- Myocardial ischemia/injury
  - Hyperacute infarction
  - Prinzmetal's angina
  - Coronary insufficiency.

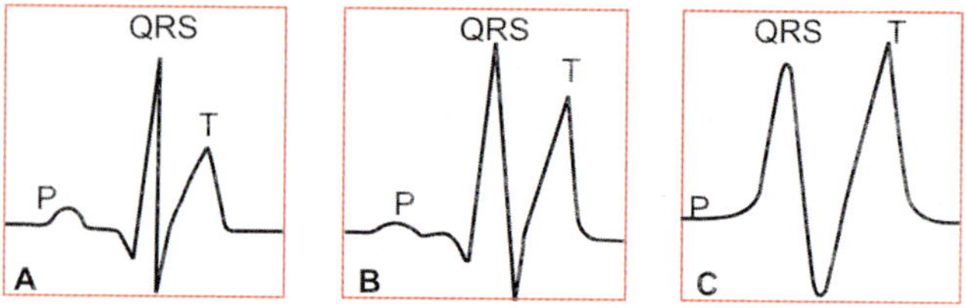

Fig. 8.8: Effects of progressively increasing hyperkalemia

A high serum potassium value is classically associated with tall T waves. The T wave of hyperkalemia is very tall, peaked, symmetrical and has a narrow base, the so called 'tented' T wave (Fig. 8.8).

Other ECG features of hyperkalemia depend upon serum potassium values and can be categorized as:

- Serum K^+ > 6.8 mEq/L

  Tall tented T waves

  Short Q-T interval

- Serum K^+ > 8.4 mEq/L

  Low/absent P waves (plus above)

- Serum K > 9.1 mEq/L

  Wide, bizarre QRS complexes

  A-V block and arrhythmias

The common causes of hyperkalemia include renal failure, adrenal insufficiency, metabolic acidosis and excessive potassium intake. The clinical importance of hyperkalemia lies in the fact that it can cause life-threatening ventricular arrhythmias.

Since hyperkalemia severe enough to cause gross ECG changes is most often due to renal failure, the clinical picture is usually that of uraemia with hypertension, fluid overload, anaemia and low urinary output.

Treatment of hyperkalemia includes elimination of dietary potassium, infusion of glucose with insulin, bicarbonate

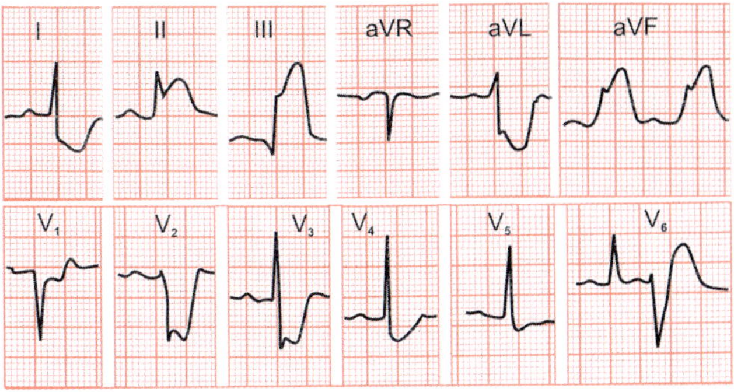

Fig. 8.9: Acute inferior wall myocardial infarction, hyperacute phase: S-T elevation in II, III, aVF; reciprocal depression in I, aVL

administration to combat acidosis, cation-exchange resins to bind potassium and haemodialysis in extreme situations.

In the hyperacute phase of myocardial infarction, there is S-T segment elevation (convex upwards) along with tall T waves, the proximal limb of the T wave blending with the elevated S-T segment (Fig. 8.9).

This phase is followed by serial evolution of ECG changes with appearance of Q waves, settling down of the S-T segment and inversion of the T waves. Because of myocardial necrosis secondary to coronary occlusion, the serum levels of cardiac enzymes (CPK, SGOT) are raised.

In a variety of angina called variant angina or Prinzmetal's angina, the basis of myocardial ischemia is not coronary thrombosis but coronary spasm. In such an ischemic episode of vasospastic angina, the ECG changes are similar to those of hyperacute phase of infarction with S-T segment elevation and tall T waves (Fig. 8.9).

The difference is that the ECG changes do not evolve serially but settle down rapidly. Q waves never appear and serum levels of cardiac enzymes are not raised as there is no myocardial necrosis.

Since the basis of Prinzmetal's angina is vasospasm, the coronary artery undergoing spasm can be predicted from the leads showing ECG changes, as depicted in Table 8.1.

Table 8.1: Relationship between location of ECG changes and coronary artery spasm

Coronary artery spasm of	*Location of ECG changes*
Left anterior descending artery	$V_1V_2V_3V_4$
Left circumflex artery	$L_IaVLV_5V_6$
Right coronary artery	$L_{II}L_{III}aVF$

The T wave may become excessively tall in the presence of coronary insufficiency. This T wave differs from the tall T wave of hyperkalemia by the fact that it is broad based and the Q-T interval is prolonged. On the other hand in hyperkalemia, the T wave is narrow based or "tented" and the Q-T interval is shortened.

CHAPTER 9

Abnormalities of the U Wave

NORMAL U WAVE

The U wave is produced by slow and late repolarization of the intraventricular Purkinje system and follows the T wave which represents repolarization of the main ventricular mass.

The normal U wave fulfills these criteria:

- It is an upright deflection
- It is much smaller than the T wave.

It is often difficult to notice the U wave but when seen, it is best appreciated in the precordial leads V_2 to V_4. The U wave is easily visible when the Q-T interval is short, being clearly separated from the T wave it follows. It is also easily visible when the heart rate is slow, being clearly separated from the P wave that follows it.

PROMINENT U WAVE

A U wave that is exaggerated and approximates the size of the T wave is considered to be a prominent U wave (Fig. 9.1). The causes of prominent U waves are:

- Hypokalemia (low serum potassium level)
- Cardiovascular drugs, e.g. digitalis, quinidine
- Psychotropic drugs, e.g. phenothiazines, tricyclics.

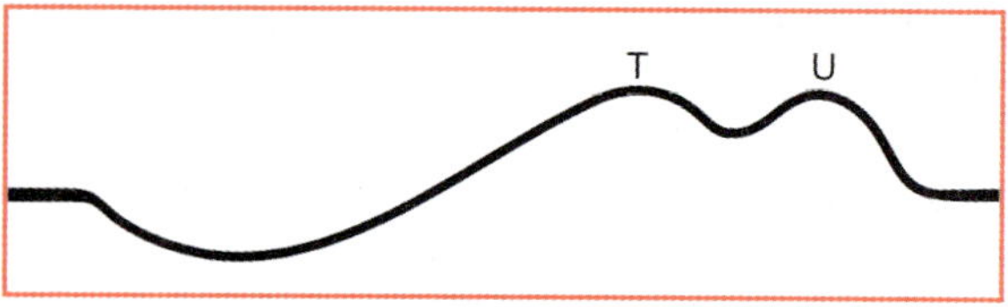

Fig. 9.1: Prominent U wave

In hypokalemia, a prominent U wave that follows a low T wave produces a 'camel-hump' effect. Alternatively, a flat T wave followed by a prominent U wave may falsely suggest prolongation of the Q-T interval while actually it is the Q-U interval that is being measured.

Certain cardiovascular therapeutic agents and psychotropic drugs can cause prominence of the U waves. Knowledge of this fact can avoid the over diagnosis of hypokalemia and Q-T interval prolongation.

INVERTED U WAVE

A U wave that is reversed in polarity is called an inverted U wave (Fig. 9.2). The causes of inverted U wave are:

- Myocardial ischemia
- Left ventricular systolic overload
- Left ventricular diastolic overload.

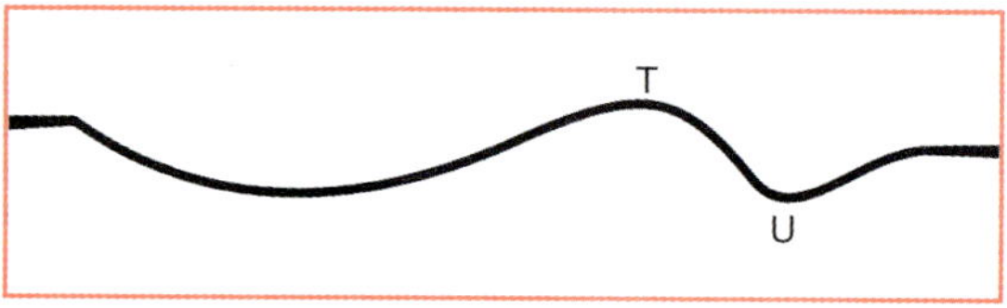

Fig. 9.2: Inverted U wave

Inversion of U waves can be taken as a sign of myocardial ischemia or ventricular strain. When due to myocardial ischemia, this is usually associated with changes in the S-T segment and T wave. Occasionally, U wave inversion may occur alone in the absence of ST-T changes.

Left ventricular overload may be systolic or diastolic. Inversion of the U wave can occur in both these conditions. This is associated with tall QRS complexes in left ventricular leads V_5, V_6, L_I and aVL. However, the strain pattern of S-T segment depression and T wave inversion is only observed in systolic overload.

CHAPTER 10

Abnormalities of the P-R Segment

All ECG deflections occur above or below a reference base-line known as the isoelectric line. The main segment of the isoelectric line intervenes between the T (or U) wave of one cardiac cycle and the P wave of the next cycle.

The portion of the isoelectric line between the termination of the P wave and the onset of the QRS complex is called the P-R segment. Normally, the P-R segment is at the same level as the main segment of the isoelectric line.

Potential abnormality of the P-R segment is depression of the P-R segment in relation to the base-line. Abnormalities of the length of the P-R segment reflect variations in the duration of the P-R interval.

P-R SEGMENT DEPRESSION

The P wave is produced by atrial depolarization. The Ta wave is produced by atrial repolarization. Normally, the Ta wave is not seen as it coincides with and lies buried in the much larger QRS complex. Prominence of the Ta wave produces depression of the P-R segment (Fig. 10.1).

The causes of P-R segment depression are:

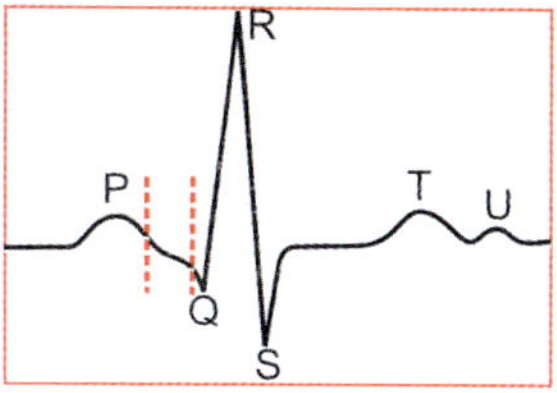

Fig. 10.1: Depressed P-R segment

- *Secondary Causes*

  Sinus tachycardia

  Atrial enlargement

- *Primary Causes*

  Acute pericarditis

  Atrial infarction

  Chest wall trauma

P-R segment depression secondary to marked sinus tachycardia has no separate clinical relevance. A depressed P-R segment alone has low sensitivity as a diagnostic criteria for atrial enlargement.

Acute pericarditis is a frequent cause of P-R segment depression and in fact, a diagnostic feature of this condition. In myocardial infarction, the P-R segment is depressed only if atrial infarction occurs. This fact is used to differentiate acute pericarditis from acute myocardial infarction since both conditions present with chest pain and ECG changes.

Depression of the P-R segment may follow trauma to the chest wall, either accidental or surgical. The P-R segment depression observed after penetrating chest wounds or cardiac surgery is due to accompanying pericarditis or atrial injury.

CHAPTER 11

Abnormalities of the S-T Segment

All ECG deflections occur above or below a reference base-line known as the isoelectric line. The main segment of the isoelectric line intervenes between the T (or U) wave of one cardiac cycle and the P wave of the next cycle.

The portion of the isoelectric line between the termination of the S wave (J point) and the onset of the T wave is called the S-T segment. Normally, the S-T segment is at the same level as the main segment of the isoelectric line.

Potential abnormalities of the S-T segment are depression or elevation of the S-T segment in relation to the base-line. Abnormalities of the length of the S-T segment reflect variation in the duration of the Q-T interval.

S-T SEGMENT DEPRESSION

Depression of the S-T segment greater than 1.0 mm in relation to the base-line constitutes significant S-T segment depression. Since depression of the S-T segment is often associated with inversion of the T wave, together they are referred to as ST-T changes.

The causes of S-T segment depression are:

NON-SPECIFIC CAUSES

- *Physiological states*

  Anxiety

  Tachycardia

  Hyperventilation

- *Extra-cardiac disorders*

  Systemic, e.g. haemorrhage, shock

  Cerebral, e.g. vascular accident

  Abdominal, e.g. pancreatitis, cholecystitis

  Respiratory, e.g. pulmonary embolism

SPECIFIC CAUSES

- *Primary abnormality*

  Pharmacological, e.g. digitalis, quinidine

  Metabolic, e.g. hypokalemia, hypothermia

  Myocardial, e.g. cardiomyopathy, myocarditis

  Ischemic, e.g. coronary insufficiency, infarction

- *Secondary abnormality*

  Ventricular hypertrophy

  Bundle branch block

  WPW syndrome

S-T segment depression lacks specificity as a diagnostic indicator. Since depression of the S-T segment can be caused by certain physiological states and non-cardiac diseases, it only highlights the importance of viewing any ECG finding in the light of clinical data.

One should be careful before diagnosing myocardial ischemia only by ECG criteria. S-T segment depression should be interpreted with caution in upper abdominal and respiratory diseases where the clinical picture may be confused with that of heart disease.

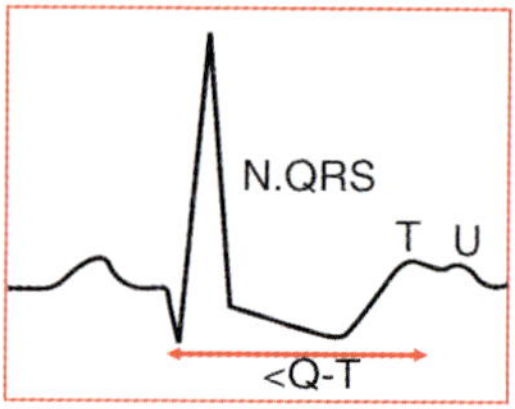

Fig. 11.1: Effects of digitalis on the P-QRS-T

Digitalis administration produces various ECG abnormalities of which S-T segment depression is an important manifestation. The depressed S-T segment either assumes a shape that is a mirror-image of the correction mark sign (√) (Fig. 11.1).

When these changes are confined to leads V_5, V_6, they indicate digitalis administration. Changes occurring in most leads are suggestive of digitalis intoxication.

Other features of digitalis administration are:

- Short Q-T interval
- Prominent U waves
- Ventricular arrhythmias

Like digitalis, quinidine also produces various abnormalities (Fig. 11.2).

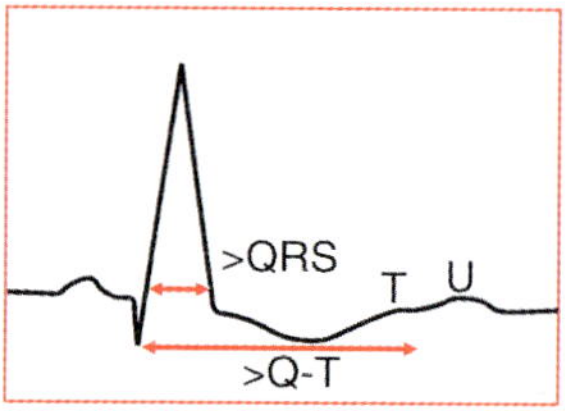

Fig. 11.2: Effects of quinidine on the P-QRS-T

Besides S-T segment depression and T wave inversion, these abnormalities are:

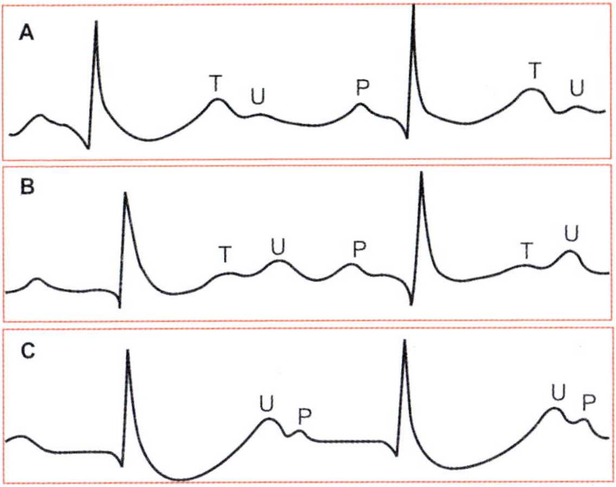

Fig. 11.3: Effects of progressively increasing hypokalemia

- Prolonged Q-T interval
- Prominent U waves
- Widened QRS complexes
- Shortened P-R interval
- Ventricular arrhythmias

Hypokalemia causes S-T segment depression (Fig. 11.3) but the more prominent abnormalities are:

- Low or flat T waves
- Prominent U waves
- Prolonged P-R interval
- Prolonged Q-U interval

Primary diseases of the myocardium such as cardiomyopathy and acute myocarditis produce S-T segment depression and T wave inversion. These changes are often associated with wide QRS complexes due to intraventricular conduction defect.

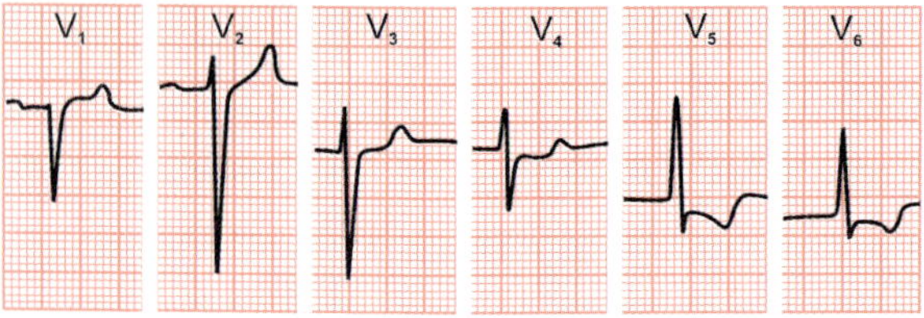

Fig. 11.4A: Lateral wall ischemic changes after angina pectoris: depression of S-T segment; inversion of T wave

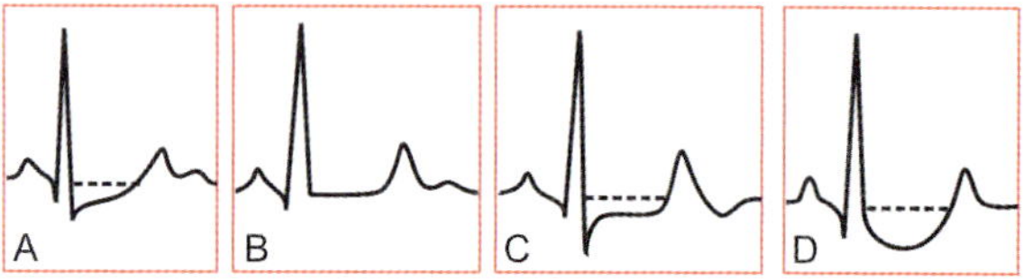

Fig. 11.4B: Various types of ST segment depression with increasing severity of myocardial ischemia
A. Isolated J point depression (upsloping S-T segment)
B. Horizontality of S-T segment (sharp ST-T junction)
C. Plane S-T depression (horizontal S-T depression)
D. Sagging depression (hammock-like S-T segment)

Clinically speaking, coronary artery disease is the most important cause of S-T segment depression. In myocardial ischemia, the degree of S-T segment depression (greater than 1 mm) generally correlates with severity of coronary insufficiency (Fig. 11.4A).

Besides being depressed, the morphology of the S-T segment associated with increasing severity of myocardial ischemia, can be classified as in Figure 11.4B.

In acute coronary insufficiency, the S-T segment acquires a coved or convex appearance. This change may be observed in several leads in contrast to localized changes seen in regional myocardial ischemia. Acute non-Q myocardial infarction may also produce an identical picture (Fig. 11.5) but with the following differences:

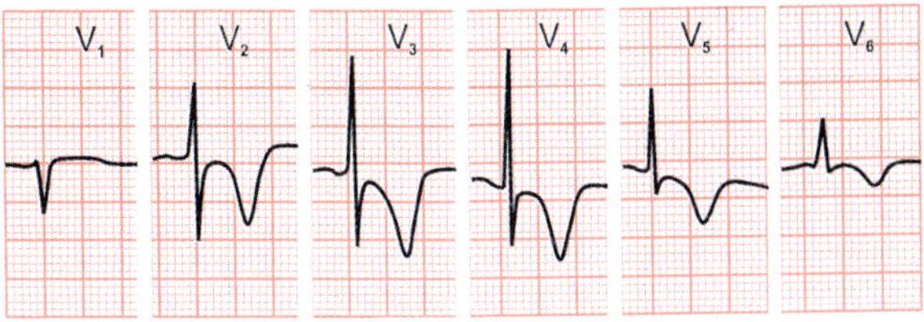

Fig. 11.5: Acute non-Q wave anterior wall myocardial infarction: convex S-T segment; symmetrical, inverted T wave

- There is history of prolonged chest pain
- Cardiac enzymes (e.g. CPK) are raised
- ST-T changes persist in serial ECGs

In acute Q-wave myocardial infarction, the ECG leads oriented towards the infarct show S-T segment elevation while the leads oriented towards the uninjured surface of the heart may reveal S-T segment depression. Such depression of the S-T segment is termed as reciprocal depression.

For instance, inferior wall myocardial infarction leads to S-T segment elevation in leads L_{II} L_{III} and aVF, while leads L_{I} and aVL show S-T segment depression (Fig. 11.6).

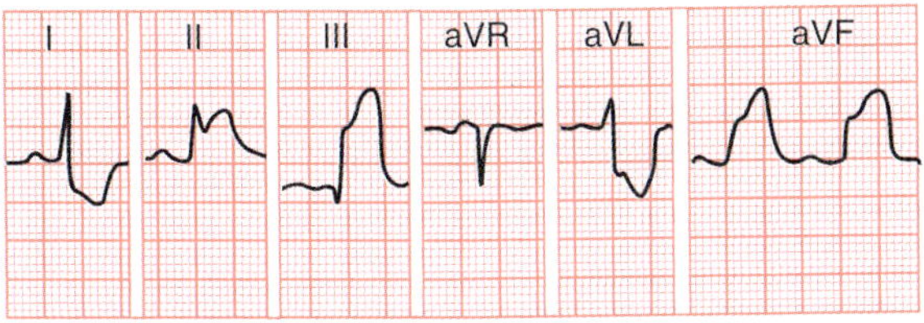

Fig. 11.6: Acute inferior wall myocardial infarction, hyperacute phase: S-T elevation in II, III, aVF; reciprocal depression in I, aVL

Depression of the S-T segment constitutes the most useful criterion for the positivity of the exercise ECG test (stress test) using a treadmill or bicycle egometer. The degree of positivity of the stress test (mild, moderate or severe) can be gauged from these parameters of S-T segment depression:

- *Degree of S-T depression*

  Greater the magnitude of S-T depression, higher is the grade of positivity of the stress test. A depression of 3 mm or more indicates severe coronary artery disease.

- *Nature of S-T depression*

  The types of S-T depression with increasing diagnostic significance are:

  Rapid upstroke of S-T segment

  Slow upstroke of S-T segment

  Horizontal ST segment depression

  Downslope ST segment depression

- *Timing of S-T depression*

  Earlier the appearance of S-T depression in the exercise period, greater is the grade of positivity of the stress test. Depression that appears in the first stage of exercise indicates greater positivity than that which appears in the third stage

- *Duration of S-T depression*

  Greater the total duration of S-T depression (exercise plus recovery period), more is the grade of positivity of the stress test. Depression that persists for upto 8 minutes of the recovery period indicates severe coronary disease.

Conditions associated with abnormal QRS morphology may also cause S-T segment depression in the leads where the QRS complex is upright. Three classical examples are ventricular hypertrophy, bundle branch block and WPW syndrome. The S-T segment depression in these conditions is secondary to an abnormality of ventricular depolarization or intraventricular conduction and is called secondary S-T segment depression.

Secondary S-T segment depression can be differentiated from primary depression of myocardial ischemia by the shape of the T wave. The T wave of ischemia is symmetrical and peaked

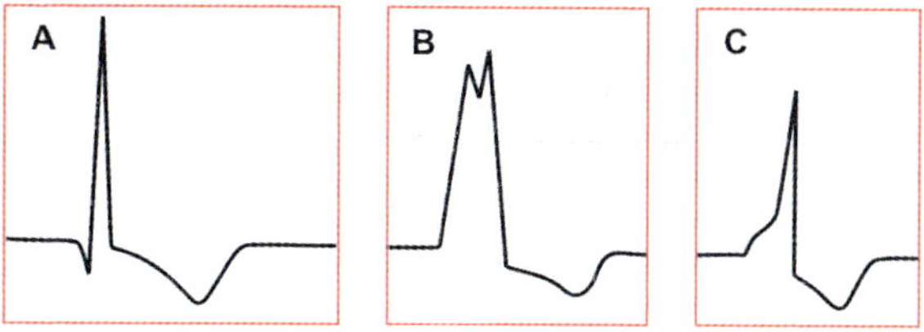

Fig. 11.7: Causes of secondary S-T depression
A. Ventricular hypertrophy
B. Bundle branch block
C. WPW syndrome

while that of secondary S-T depression is asymmetrical and blunt (Fig. 11.7).

S-T SEGMENT ELEVATION

Elevation of the S-T segment exceeding 1 mm in relation to the base-line constitutes significant S-T segment elevation. The causes of S-T segment elevation are:

- Coronary artery disease
    - Myocardial infarction
    - Prinzmetal's angina
    - Dressler's syndrome
- Acute pericarditis
- Ventricular aneurysm
- Early repolarization.

Acute myocardial infarction is the most common and clinically the most significant cause of S-T segment elevation. In the hyperacute phase of infarction, the elevated S-T segment slopes upwards to blend smoothly with the proximal limb of the T wave. In this stage, the T wave is upright and the Q wave is not observed. In the evolved phase, the elevated S-T segment

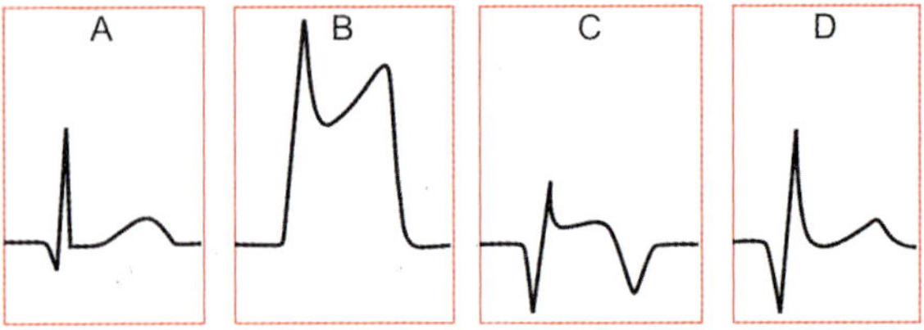

Fig. 11.8: Phases of acute myocardial infarction
A. Normal QRS-T complex
B. Hyperacute phase
C. Fully evolved phase
D. Stabilized phase

becomes convex upwards, the T wave gets symmetrically inverted, the Q wave appears and there is loss of R wave height (Fig. 11.8).

The leads which show S-T segment elevation in myocardial infarction depend upon the location of the infarct and can be expressed as given in Table 11.1.

Table 11.1: Location of infarction determined from ECG leads

S-T elevation in	*Location of infarction*
V_1 to V_4	Anteroseptal
V_1, V_2	Septal
V_3, V_4	Anterior
L_I, aVL	High lateral
V_5-V_6 L_I aVL	Lateral
V_3-V_6 L_I aVL	Anterolateral
V_1-V_6 L_I aVL	Extensive anterior
L_{II} L_{III} avF	Inferior
V_3R V_4R	Right ventricular

Besides S-T segment elevation, other electrocardiographic features of myocardial infarction are:

- Symmetrical T wave inversion
- Appearance of Q wave
- Loss of R wave height
- Regional location of changes
- Reciprocal S-T depression in other leads
- Arrhythmias and conduction defects
- Serial evolution of ECG changes

In Prinzmetal's angina, the ECG changes are very similar to those of the hyperacute phase of myocardial infarction with the following differences:

- ECG changes resolve rapidly and do not evolve serially
- Serum levels of cardiac enzymes (e.g. CPK) are normal.

The basis of Prinzmetal's angina is coronary spasm and not coronary thrombosis as in the case of myocardial infarction. Coronary spasm may be provoked by injection of intracoronary ergonovine. The coronary artery undergoing spasm can be predicted from the leads showing S-T elevation as shown in Table 11.2.

Table 11.2: Relationship between location of S-T elevation and coronary artery spasm

S-T elevation in	*Coronary artery spasm of*
V_1 V_2 V_3 V_4	Left anterior descending artery
V_5 V_6 L_1 avL	Left circumflex artery
L_{II} L_{III} avF	Right coronary artery

Besides acute myocardial infaction, another frequent cause of S-T segment elevation is acute pericarditis. Since both these

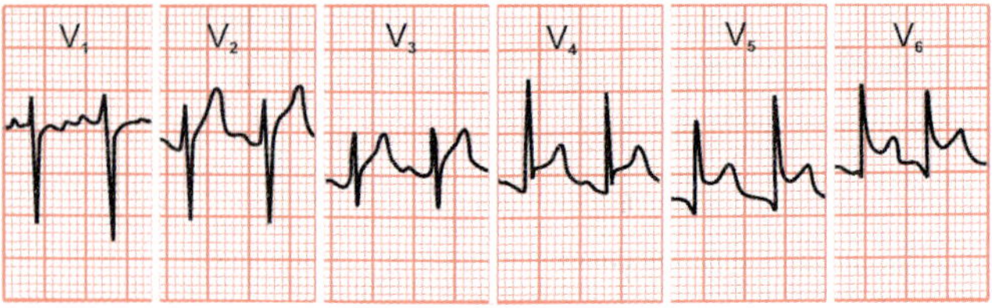

Fig. 11.9: Acute pericarditis: concave upward S-T segment elevation

conditions are associated with chest pain, given the more serious nature of myocardial infarction, it is extremely important to differentiate them.

Electrocardiographic features of acute pericarditis, as different from those of acute myocardial infarction are:

- S-T segment elevation is concave upwards (Fig.11.9)
- S-T elevation is observed in nearly all leads
- T waves invert after S-T returns to base-line
- Q waves do not appear
- R wave height is maintained
- P-R segment is depressed
- There is no reciprocal S-T segment depression
- Sinus tachycardia is almost invariably present
- Arrhythmias and conduction defects are unusual
- ECG changes do not evolve but resolve rapidly.

During, the resolving phase of acute myocardial infarction, occasionally, there may be re-elevation of the S-T segment for which three explanations may be offered.

- Firstly, it may be due to reinfarction with re-elevation of cardiac enzymes requiring intensive treatment.
- Secondly, it may represent coronary vasospasm, the significance of which is similar to that of Prinzmetal's angina.

- Finally, S-T segment re-elevation may be due to the post-infarction syndrome or Dressler's syndrome.

The specific features of Dressler' syndrome are:

- Elevation of S-T segment without reciprocal depression
- Precordial pain increasing on inspiration
- Fever and tachycardia are often present
- Raised ESR but normal cardiac enzymes
- Appearance of pleuro-pericardial rub
- Responsiveness to steroid therapy

A picture similar to that in Dressler's syndrome may be observed in the post-cardiotomy syndrome that follows cardiac surgery, chest wall trauma or pacemaker implant.

Any survivor of myocardial infarction in whom the typical pattern of the evolved phase of infarction persists for three months or longer after acute attack, should be suspected to have developed a ventricular aneurysm.

However, this ECG sign has a low sensitivity for the diagnosis of an aneurysm. The presence of a ventricular aneurysm has to be confirmed by echocardiography.

There exists a benign but often alarming electrocardiographic entity that presents with S-T segment elevation and an entirely normal clinical profile. It is known as the "early repolarization" syndrome.

There is an early uptake of the S-T segment before the descending limb of the R wave has reached the baseline. This causes an initial slur on the S-T segment known as the J wave.

It represents early repolarization of a portion of the myocardium, before the entire myocardium has been depolarized (Fig. 11.10).

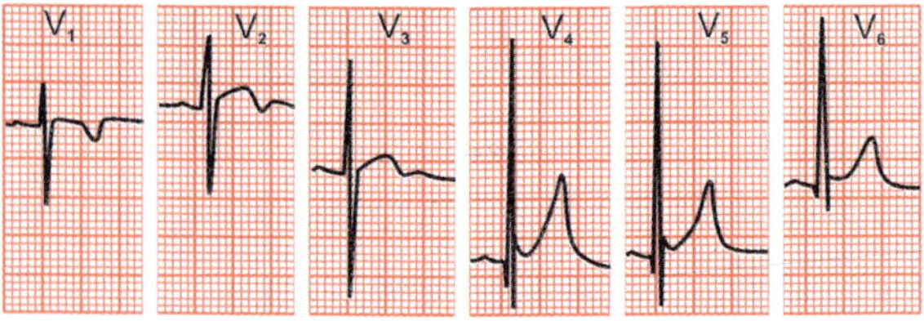

Fig. 11.10: ECG features of early repolarization syndrome
a. tall R waves in leads V_4 to V_6
b. deep and narrow initial q waves
c. concave-upward ST segment elevation
d. initial slur on ST segment; the J wave
e. tall and upright symmetrical T waves

The clinical features of early repolarization syndrome are:

- subject is a young black male
- he is healthy and of athletic built
- he is active and free from symptoms
- the clinical evaluation is entirely normal
- ST segment returns to baseline after exercise.

12 CHAPTER

Abnormalities of the P-R Interval

NORMAL P-R INTERVAL

The P-R interval is measured on the horizontal axis from the onset of the P wave to the beginning of the QRS complex, irrespective of whether it begins with a Q wave or R wave. The width of the P wave is included in the length of P-R interval.

Since the P wave represents atrial depolarization and the QRS complex represents ventricular depolarization, the P-R interval is a measure of the atrioventricular (AV) conduction time. The AV conduction time includes the time taken for atrial depolarization, the conduction delay in the A-V node and the time taken for an impulse to traverse the intraventricular conduction system before ventricular depolarization begins.

Since the conduction delay in the A-V node is the major fraction of the P-R interval, the length of P-R interval is a measure of the duration of A-V nodal delay.

The normal P-R interval in adults ranges from 0.12 to 0.20 sec depending upon the heart rate. It is longer at slow heart rates and shorter at fast heart rates. The P-R interval is slightly shorter in children, the upper limit being 0.18 sec. It is slightly longer in the elderly, the upper limit being 0.22 sec.

Potential abnormalities of the P-R interval are:

- Prolonged P-R interval
- Shortened P-R interval
- Variable P-R interval

PROLONGED P-R INTERVAL

A P-R interval that exceeds 0.20 sec in adults and 0.18 sec in children is taken as prolonged. Since the P-R interval reflects atrioventricular conduction time, a prolonged P-R interval indicates increased A-V nodal conduction delay or first degree atrioventricular (AV) block (Fig. 12.1).

The causes of prolonged P-R interval are:

- Vagal dominance in athletes
- Acute rheumatic fever or diphtheria
- Coronary artery disease with fascicular block
- Drugs acting on the A-V node, e.g. digitalis, beta-blockers, calcium-channel blockers.

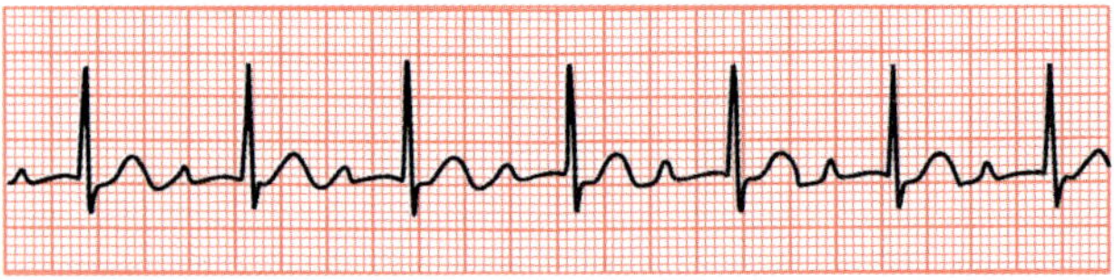

Fig.12.1: Prolonged P-R interval: first-degree A-V block

Clinical Relevance of Prolonged P-R Interval

P-R interval prolongation is normally observed in vagotonic individuals such as athletes. It is also a normal effect of vagal stimulation, e.g. carotid sinus massage and sympathetic blockade, e.g. beta-blocker administration

A prolonged P-R interval is one of the diagnostic criteria of acute rheumatic fever and indicates carditis. Similarly, a prolonged P-R interval in diphtheria indicates myocarditis.

P-R interval prolongation is usual with cardiovascular drugs that act on the A-V node and delay A-V conduction.Examples are digitalis, verapamil, diltiazem, propranolol and metoprolol.

Prolongation of the P-R interval in the presence of bundle branch of block indicates that atrioventricular conduction down the unblocked bundle branch is also delayed. Since such patients are likely to develop complete A-V block, they may require prophylactic cardiac pacing.

SHORTENED P-R INTERVAL

A P-R interval that is less than 0.12 sec is considered short. Since P-R interval reflects atrioventricular conduction time, a short P-R interval indicates decreased A-V nodal delay.

The causes of shortened P-R interval are:

- A-V nodal or junctional rhythm
- WPW syndrome with pre-excitation
- Drugs that hasten A-V conduction, e.g. atropine, quinidine.

Clinical Relevance of Shortened P-R Interval

If a cardiac rhythm originates from the A-V nodal area (junctional rhythm), the ventricles are activated in the normal sequence but the atria are activated retrogradely, that is, from below upwards. Since the atria are activated nearly simultaneously with the ventricles, the P waves just precede, just follow or are merged in the QRS complexes. When the P waves just precede the QRS complexes, they are associated with a short P-R interval (Fig. 12.2).

A junctional rhythm at its inherent discharge rate of 40-60 beats per minute constitutes a junctional escape rhythm while a junctional rhythm at an enhanced rate of 60-100 beats per minute constitutes a junctional tachycardia.

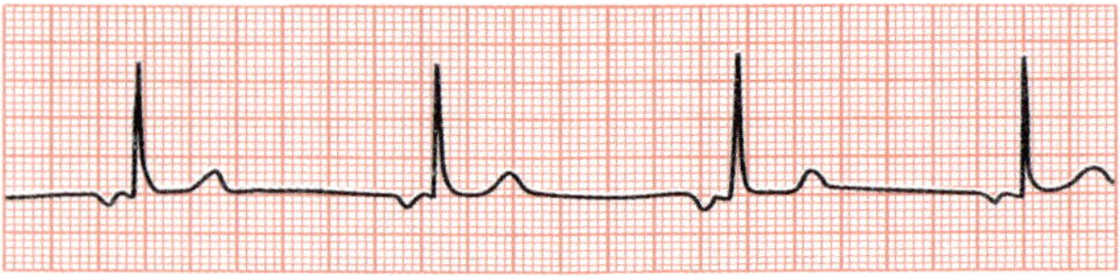

Fig. 12.2: Shortened P-R interval: junctional rhythm

The WPW syndrome is an entity in which an accessory pathway or by-pass tract called the bundle of Kent connects the atrial to the ventricular myocardium without passing through the A-V node. Conduction of impulses down this tract results in premature ventricular activation called pre-excitation, since the A-V node is by-passed. This results in a short P-R interval.

The P-R interval is prolonged in vagotonic individuals and with vagal stimulation. Conversely, the P-R interval is shortened with vagolytic drugs, e.g. atropine and drugs with anticholinergic effects, e.g. quinidine.

VARIABLE P-R INTERVAL

During any rhythm, a changing P-R interval on a beat-to-beat basis is designated as variable P-R interval. Normally, atrial activation (P wave) is followed by ventricular activation (QRS complex) with an identical intervening P-R interval in all beats, thus establishing fixed relationship between them.

If atrial and ventricular activation occur independent of each other and not sequentially, or if the extent of A-V nodal conduction delay varies from beat-to-beat, the P-R interval is variable.

The causes of variable P-R interval are:

- Type I, second-degree A-V block
- Junctional pacemaker rhythm
- Complete, third-degree A-V block
- Wandering pacemaker rhythm
- Multifocal atrial tachycardia.

13 CHAPTER

Abnormalities of the Q-T Interval

NORMAL Q-T INTERVAL

The Q-T interval is measured on the horizontal axis from the onset of the Q wave to the termination of the T wave (not the U wave). The duration of the QRS complex, the length of the S-T segment and the width of the T wave are included in the measurement of the Q-T interval.

Since the QRS duration represents ventricular depolarization time and the T wave width represents ventricular repolarization time the Q-T interval is a measure of the total duration of ventricular electrical activity.

The normal Q-T interval is in the range of 0.35 to 0.43 sec or 0.39 ± 0.04 sec. The normal Q-T interval depends upon three variables namely age, sex and heart rate.

The Q-T interval tends to be shorter in young individuals and longer in the elderly. It is slightly shorter in females, the upper limit being 0.42 sec. The Q-T interval shortens at fast heart rates and lengthens at slow heart rates.

Therefore, for proper interpretation, the Q-T interval must be corrected for the heart rate. The corrected Q-T interval is known as the Q-Tc interval. The Q-Tc interval is determined using the formula:

$$\text{Q-Tc} = \frac{\text{Q-T}}{\sqrt{\text{R-R}}}$$

Q-T is the measured Q-T interval

$\sqrt{R\text{-}R}$ is square-root of R-R interval

When the R - R interval is 25 mm or 1 sec (25 × 0.04 sec = 1 sec), the value of $\sqrt{R\text{-}R}$ is 1 and the Q-Tc is equal to the Q-T interval. This occurs at a heart rate of 60 beats/min.

Potential abnormalities of the Q-T interval are:

- Shortened Q-T interval
- Prolonged Q-T interval

SHORTENED Q-T INTERVAL

A corrected Q-T interval (Q-Tc interval) less than 0.35 sec is considered short. The causes of a shortened Q-Tc interval are:

- Hyperkalemia
- Hypercalcemia
- Digitalis effect

Clinical Relevance of Shortened Q-T Interval

Hyperkalemia shortens the Q-T interval and is associated with tall T waves, wide QRS complexes and diminished P waves. Hypercalcemia also shortens the Q-T interval but there are no changes in the morphology of the QRS deflection or T wave (Fig.13.1).

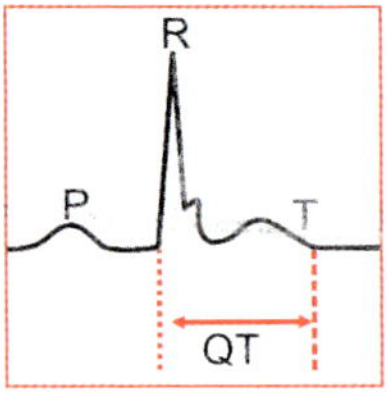

Fig. 13.1: Shortened Q-T interval: hypercalcemia

A short Q-T interval with S-T segment depression and T wave inversion suggests digitalis effect. Quinidine-like drugs also produce ST-T changes but the Q-T interval is prolonged.

PROLONGED Q-T INTERVAL

A corrected Q-T interval (Q-Tc interval) greater than 0.43 sec is considered prolonged. The causes of a prolonged Q-Tc interval can be classified as:

- Congenital causes

  Congenital Q-T prolongation

  Mitral valve prolapse syndrome

- Acquired causes

  Electrolyte deficiency, e.g. calcium, magnesium

  Antiarrhythmic drugs, e.g. quinidine, amiodarone

  Coronary disease, e.g. myocardial infarction

  Acute myocarditis, e.g. viral myocarditis, rheumatic fever

  Intracranial event, e.g. head injury, haemorrhage

  Bradyarrhythmias, e.g. A-V block, sinus bradycardia.

Hypocalcemia produces true prolongation of the Q-T interval without any alteration of the S-T segment or T wave (Fig. 13.2).

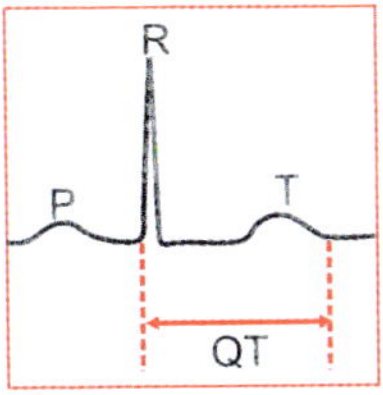

Fig. 13.2: Prolonged Q-T interval: hypocalcemia

In hypokalemia, the T wave is flattened and the prominent U wave may be mistaken for the T wave. This may falsely suggest prolongation of the Q-T interval, whereas it is actually the Q-U interval. Hypokalemia, therefore, causes pseudo-prolongation of the Q-T interval (Fig. 13.3).

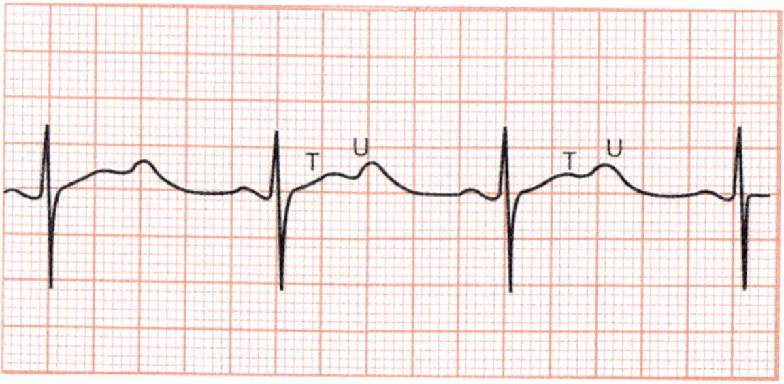

Fig. 13.3: Pseudo-prolongation of the Q-T interval: hypokalemia

Antiarrhythmic drugs such as quinidine, procainamide and amiodarone can prolong the Q-T interval. They also cause widening of the QRS complex which if exceeds 25 percent of base-line, is an indication for withdrawing the culprit drug.

Since Q-T interval prolongation predisposes to arrhythmias, this is one way to explain the arrhythmia enhancing property or proarrhythmic effect of antiarrhythmic drugs.

The clinical importance of Q-T interval prolongation lies in the fact that it predisposes to a typical type of polymorphic ventricular arrhythmia known as “Torsade de pointes” which literally means “torsion of points”.

This term explains the morphology of the ventricular tachycardia which consists of polymorphic QRS complexes that keep changing in amplitude and direction. The polymorphic QRS complexes give the appearance of torsion or twisting of points around the isoelectric line.

CHAPTER 14

Premature Beats Interrupting Regular Sinus Rhythm

PREMATURE BEATS

Premature beats are impulses that arise due to the premature discharge of an ectopic focus located outside the normal pacemaker. They are also known as premature contractions, premature complexes or simply extrasystole.

According to focus of origin, premature beats are classified as:

- Atrial premature beats
- Junctional premature beats
- Ventricular premature beats.

Atrial and junctional premature complexes are together referred to as supraventricular premature beats.

ATRIAL PREMATURE COMPLEX

An atrial premature complex (APC) (Fig. 14.1) is recognized by the following features:

- Premature inscription of an upright P wave, earlier than the expected sinus P wave.
- Abnormal morphology of the premature P wave due to ectopic focus of origin.

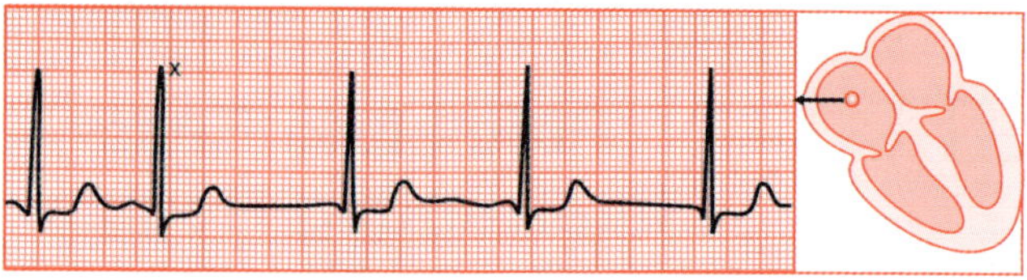

Fig. 14.1: Atrial premature beat: ectopic P wave, narrow QRS, incomplete compensatory pause

- Normal morphology of the QRS complex that follows it, since ventricular conduction is normal.
- Compensatory pause after the APC due to momentary suppression of S-A node automaticity.

Occasionally, two variations of APCs may be observed

- *Blocked APC* A very premature APC may find the A-V node still refractory to ventricular conduction and may consequently get blocked. Such an APC inscribes a P wave that deforms the T wave of the preceding beat, is not followed by a QRS complex but is followed by a compensatory pause.
- *APC with aberrant ventricular conduction* Most often, the QRS complex of the APC is normal in morphology. However, if the APC finds one of the bundle branches still refractory to ventricular conduction, it inscribes a wide QRS complex or bundle branch block pattern. This is known as aberrant ventricular conduction of the APC.

APCs alternating with sinus impulses constitute a bigeminal rhythm (extrasystolic atrial bigeminy) while a series of three or more successive APCs constitute an atrial tachycardia. Frequent APCs arising from different atrial foci constitute a multifocal atrial tachycardia.

JUNCTIONAL PREMATURE COMPLEX

A junctional premature complex (JPC) (Fig. 14.2) is very similar to an APC but with these differences:

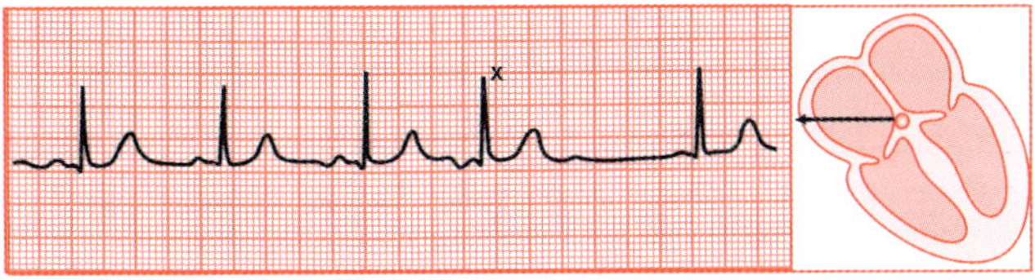

Fig. 14.2: Junctional premature beat: inverted P wave, narrow QRS, incomplete compensatory pause

- The P wave of the JPC if seen, is inverted because of retrograde atrial activation.
- The P wave just precedes, just follows or is merged in the QRS complex because of near simultaneous atrial and ventricular activation.

Since, both atrial and junctional premature complexes have a somewhat similar clinical relevance and are managed in the same way, their differentiation is often futile and they are together referred to as supraventricular premature complexes.

VENTRICULAR PREMATURE COMPLEX

A ventricular premature complex (VPC) (Fig. 14.3) is recognized by the following features:

- Premature inscription of a QRS complex earlier than the next expected sinus beat.

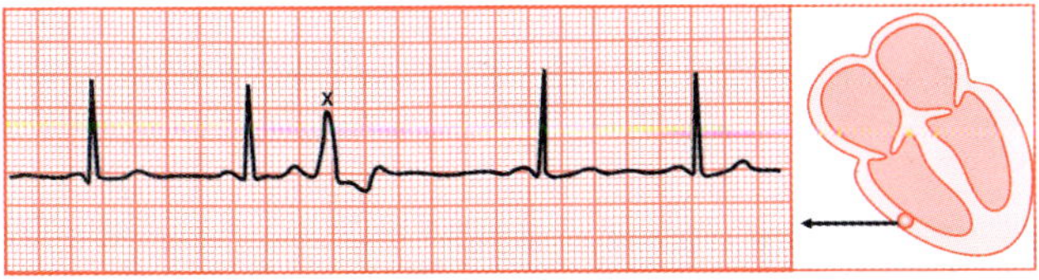

Fig. 14.3: Ventricular premature beat: absent P wave, wide QRS, complete compensatory pause

- Wide and bizarre morphology of the QRS complex due to slow activation of the ventricles.
- Bizarre QRS complex is not preceded by a P wave because of ventricular origin of the beat. A sinus P wave even if it occurs independently, is not visible as it is buried in the wide QRS complex.
- Compensatory pause after the VPC. When a VPC is inscribed, a sinus beat that was to occur around that time is missed but the next sinus beat is inscribed as usual. This is expressed as a compensatory pause after the VPC. The compensatory pause after a VPC is complete, that is, it fully compensates for the prematurity of the VPC. This is in contrast to an APC where the compensatory pause is incomplete and the next sinus beat is only somewhat delayed.

On the basis of their occurrence, VPCs can be qualified as:

- VPCs of different morphology and coupling intervals (between VPC and preceding sinus beat) are called multifocal VPCs.
- VPC occurring late in the diastolic period of the preceding sinus beat (long coupling interval), just about when the next sinus beat is due, is called an end-diastolic VPC.
- VPC that is so premature (very short coupling interval) that it is imposed upon the T wave of the preceding sinus impulse, exhibits the R-on-T phenomenon (Fig. 14.4).

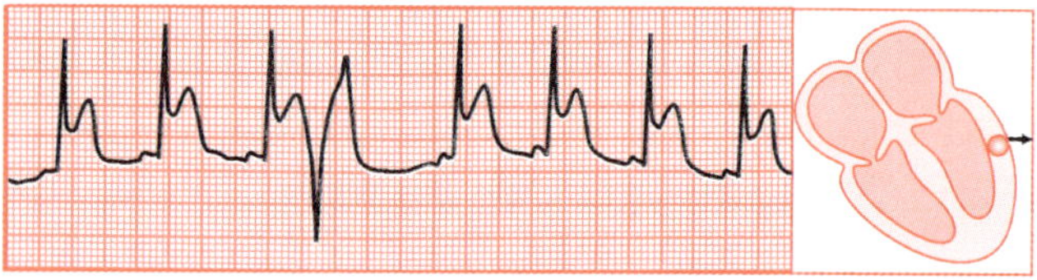

Fig. 14.4: Ventricular ectopic beat exhibiting R-on-T phenomenon: VPC deforming the T wave of the preceding sinus beat

- VPC during a slow rhythm, that does not allow any sinus beat to be missed and is not followed by a compensatory pause, is called an interpolated VPC.
- VPCs alternating with sinus beats constitute a bigeminal rhythm (extrasystolic ventricular bigeminy) (Fig. 14.5). VPCs after every two sinus beats represent trigeminy and after every third sinus beat constitute quadrigeminy.

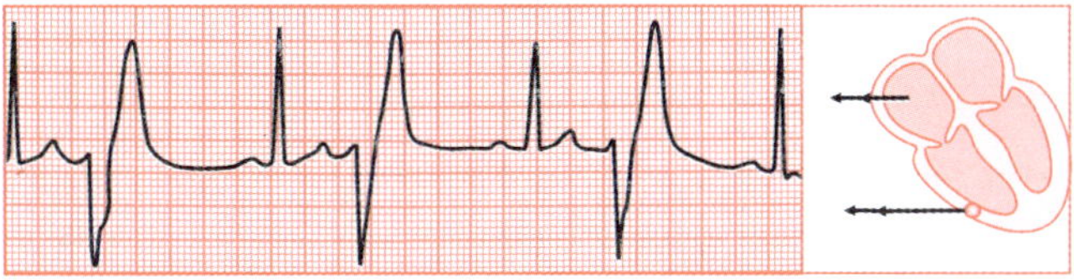

Fig. 14.5: Extrasystolic ventricular bigeminy: ectopic beats alternating with sinus beats

- A pair of successive VPCs form a couplet (Fig. 14.6) and three or more consecutive VPCs constitute a ventricular tachycardia.

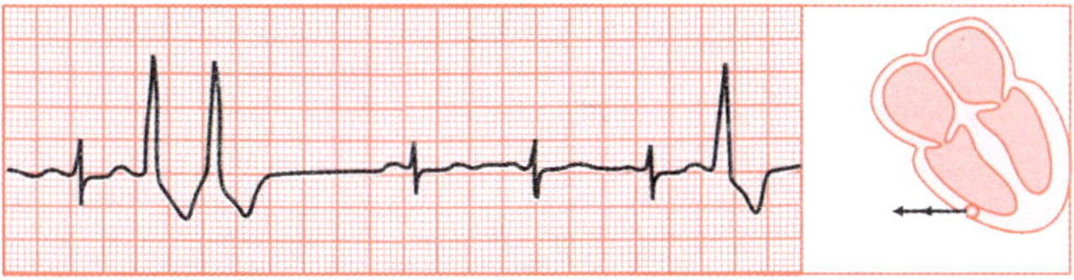

Fig. 14.6: Couplet of ventricular ectopic beats: two VPCs occurring in succession

A VPC is quite different in morphology from an APC, the former having a wide and bizarre QRS complex while the latter possessing a narrow QRS complex. Their differentiation assumes importance only if an APC conducts aberrantly to the ventricles and inscribes a wide QRS complex.

An APC with aberrant ventricular conduction can be differentiated from a true VPC by the following features:

- Preceding P wave
- Triphasic QRS contour
- Incomplete compensatory pause.

Clinical Relevance of Premature Complexes

Supraventricular Premature Complexes

Atrial premature complexes (APCs) are common even in normal persons and occur due to these causes:

- Emotional stress or physical exercise
- Smoking or high intake of tea/coffee
- Drugs, e.g. salbutamol, theophylline
- Metabolic causes, e.g. hypoxia, acidosis.

Junctional premature complexes (JPCs) are less common than APCs and are less likely to occur in normal persons. In other words, their presence is more indicative of heart disease.

Cardiac causes of APCs and JPCs are:

- Rheumatic carditis
- Digitalis toxicity
- Myocardial infarction
- Pericarditis
- Thyrotoxicosis
- Cardiac surgery.

Although APCs may be asymptomatic, the most common symptoms due to them are palpitations and sensation of "missed beats". JPCs cause similar symptoms but additionally produce neck-pulsation because of synchronous atrial and ventricular contraction or atrial contraction during A-V valve closure.

Treatment of supraventricular premature complexes is generally not required especially if they are asymptomatic and not associated with organic heart disease. Management is indicated if premature beats are frequent enough to produce symptoms or if they trigger tachyarrhythmias such as supraventricular tachycardia or atrial flutter.

The first step in management is avoidance of precipitating factors such as stress, vigorous exercise, smoking, beverage consumption and adrenergic drugs. Addition of a mild sedative may be useful in some patients. The next step is treatment of any underlying cardiac condition if present. This includes withdrawal of digitalis, treatment of rheumatic fever, control of thyrotoxicosis and management of ischemia.

If premature beats are frequent, low doses of beta-blockers or diltiazem are effective in controlling the ventricular rate. Propranolol may be the drug of choice in the management of premature beats caused by anxiety, adrenergic drugs and other catecholamine excess states. Amiodarone is quite effective in suppressing the ectopic atrial focus.

Ventricular Premature Complexes

Ventricular premature complexes (VPCs) can occur even in normal individuals although they are more often due to organic heart disease.

Causes of VPCs in normal persons are:

- Emotional stress or physical exercise
- Smoking or high intake of tea/coffee
- Drugs, e.g. sympathomimetics, theophylline
- Anxiety neurosis or thyrotoxicosis

Cardiac conditions where VPCs are observed are:

- *Coronary Artery Disease*

    Ischemia

    Infarction

    Reperfusion

- *Congestive heart failure*
  - Hypertension
  - Cardiomyopathy
  - Myocarditis
  - Ventricular aneurysm
- *Mitral Valve Prolapse Syndrome*
- *Digitalis Treatment/Intoxication*
- *Cardiac Surgery or Catheterization.*

VPCs that meet the following criteria are considered to be "dangerous" or "malignant" VPCs.

- Occurring frequently (6 or more beats/min)
- In showers with runs of ventricular tachycardia
- In couplets or VPCs in bigeminal rhythm
- With short coupling interval (R-on-T)
- More than 0.14 sec wide, bizarre or multifocal
- Associated with serious organic heart disease and left ventricular dysfunction.

Severity of ventricular ectopy can be classified on the basis of Lown's classification, as given in Table 14.1.

Table 14.1: Lown's classification of ventricular ectopy

Category	*Degree of ectopy*
Class 0	No ectopy
Class 1	Less than 30/hour
Class 2	More than 30/hour
Class 3	Multiform VPCs
Class 4A	Couplets
Class 4B	Runs of 3 or more
Class 5	R-on-T phenomenon

A VPC that occurs very prematurely (very short coupling interval) superimposes on the T wave of the preceding sinus beat and is said to exhibit the 'R-on-T' phenomenon. This represents the occurrence of ventricular stimulation during the vulnerable phase or period of supernormal excitability and is likely to precipitate ventricular fibrillation.

The 'R-on-T' phenomenon is observed in:

- VPCs after acute myocardial infarction
- VPCs with underlying Q-T interval prolongation
- Electrical cardioversion during digitalis therapy
- Very premature stimuli during artificial pacing.

VPCs may be asymptomatic or associated with palpitations and sensation of "missed beats". Awareness of VPCs is due to the post-VPC compensatory pause and increased force of contraction of the beat following the VPC.

Neck pulsations may be felt due to atrial systole occurring with a closed tricuspid valve as the atria and ventricles are activated almost synchronously by the VPC.

Management of VPCs is governed by:

- Symptoms produced by premature beats
- Presence or absence of organic heart disease
- Nature and severity of ventricular ectopy

Few isolated asymptomatic VPCs, in the absence of heart disease, are mostly left alone. If they are symptomatic, a search for aetiological factors must be made and they should be corrected adequately.

Such measures include:

- Alleviating anxiety and stress
- Reduction of smoking and beverages
- Withdrawal of adrenergic drugs
- Management of digitalis intoxication

- Treatment of congestive heart failure
- Management of myocardial ischemia.

Antiarrhythmic drugs may be used in symptomatic patients with organic heart disease and significant ventricular ectopy in whom correction of precipitating factors does not suffice.

Beta-blockers like propranolol and metoprolol are the drugs of choice for treatment of VPCs associated with anxiety, physical exercise, mitral valve prolapse or thyrotoxicosis.

Lidocaine and amiodarone are the drugs of choice for VPCs after myocardial infarction, cardiac surgery or catheterization.

When a patient of congestive heart failure on digitalis develops significant VPCs, it has to be decided on clinical grounds whether digitalis should be continued to manage the heart failure or withdrawn in view of drug intoxication.

If digitalis is to be withdrawn, the antiarrhythmic drug of choice for digitalis induced VPCs is phenytoin sodium which should be used in conjunction with standard therapy of digitalis intoxication.

Antiarrhythmic drugs may be used for control of VPCs but before initiating treatment with these drugs, the following issues need to be addressed to:

- Inappropriate drug usage, when the cause and effect relationship of VPCs to fatal ventricular arrhythmias has not been established.
- Proarrhythmic effect of these drugs with increased likelihood of other tachyarrhythmias.
- Potential systemic side-effects associated with long-term antiarrhythmic therapy.

CHAPTER 15

Pauses During Sinus Rhythm

PAUSES IN RHYTHM

A pause during normal regular sinus rhythm is a brief period of electrical inactivity on the ECG graph between successive beats, due to delay in onset of the next scheduled beat. A pause produces a larger gap between two successive beats than that seen in other parts of the rhythm.

The causes of pauses are:

- Premature beats
- Sinoatrial block
- Atrioventricular block

PAUSE AFTER PREMATURE BEAT

A premature beat, whether supraventricular or ventricular, is followed by a pause that compensates for its prematurity. This is known as the compensatory pause.

In the case of a supraventricular premature beat, there is a momentary suppression of S-A node automaticity so that the next sinus beat is somewhat delayed. This results in an incomplete compensatory pause, that is, the interval between the beat preceding and following the premature beat is less than twice the R-R interval between two successive sinus beats.

In the case of ventricular premature beat, one sinus beat after the premature beat fails to activate the already depolarized ventricles while the second sinus beat occurs as usual. This results in a complete compensatory pause, which fully compensates for the prematurity of the ectopic beat. In other words, the interval between the beat preceding and that following the premature beat is exactly twice the R-R interval between two successive sinus beats.

PAUSE AFTER BLOCKED PREMATURE BEAT

A very premature atrial ectopic beat may find the A-V node refractory to ventricular conduction, having already been traversed by the preceding sinus beat. Therefore, it gets blocked in the A-V node and fails to inscribe a QRS complex. Nevertheless, the ectopic P wave of the premature beat deforms the T wave of the preceding sinus beat and is followed by a pause.

This premature ectopic P wave is the key to the differentiation of a non-conducted atrial premature beat from a pause due to sinoatrial block or atrioventricular block.

PAUSE DUE TO SINOATRIAL BLOCK

Sinoatrial block refers to an interference with the propagation of an impulse from the sinus node to the surrounding atrial myocardium, resulting in a delay or omission of an atrial response.

There are three degrees of sinoatrial block:

- **1° S-A block** First-degree S-A block cannot be diagnosed from the ECG as there are no dropped beats. Electrophysiological study reveals slow sinoatrial conduction.
- **2° S-A block** In second-degree S-A block, there is intermittent dropping of one more beats. In fact, an entire beat (P wave with QRS complex) is dropped as neither atrial nor ventricular activation occurs (Fig. 15.1).

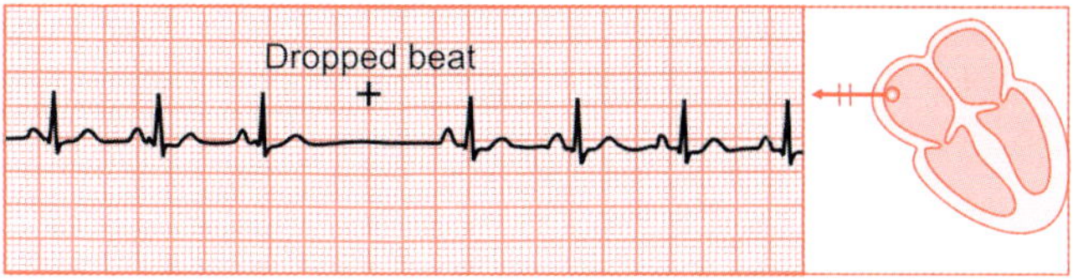

Fig. 15.1: Dropped beat due to second-degree sinoatrial block

If every second beat is dropped, that is, in a period of time when there should be 2 beats but there is only one beat, it is called 2:1 S-A block. If every third beat is dropped, that is, 2 beats occur in a period of time when there should be 3 beats, it is called 3:2 S-A block.

- **3° S-A block** This is also known as complete S-A block, sinus arrest or atrial standstill (Fig. 15.2). In third-degree S-A block, there is a prolonged period of electrical inactivity or asystole following which either an escape rhythm from a subsidiary pacemaker takes over or prolonged asystole results in cardiac arrest.

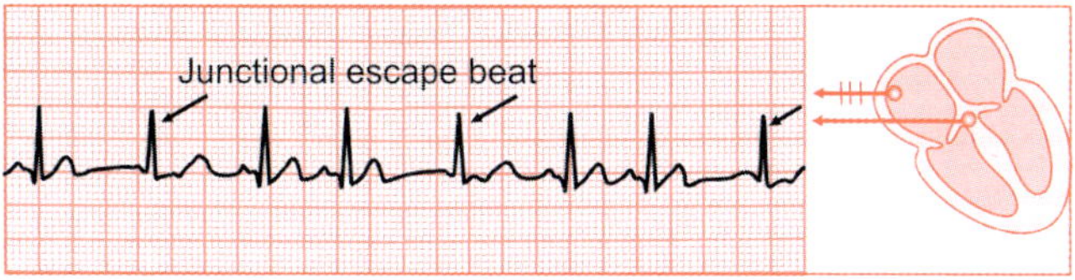

Fig. 15.2: Sinus arrest followed by a junctional escape beat

Second-degree S-A block needs to be differentiated from two other conditions.

- A non-conducted atrial ectopic beat also results in a pause resembling S-A block. However, the non-conducted ectopic beat inscribes a premature ectopic P wave that superimposes on the T wave of the preceding sinus beat.
- A second-degree atrioventricular block (A-V block) also results in missing of a beat but in that case, the P wave is inscribed normally and only the QRS complex is missing.

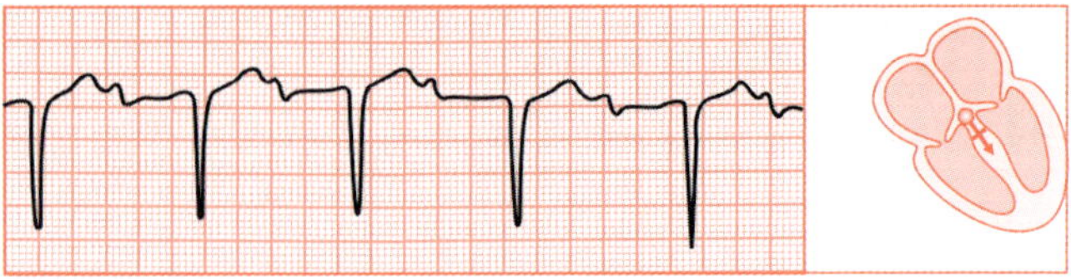

Fig. 15.3: First-degree A-V block: prolonged P-R interval

PAUSE DUE TO ATRIOVENTRICULAR BLOCK

Atrioventricular block refers to an interference with the propagation of an impulse from the atria to the ventricles, resulting in a delay or omission, of a ventricular reponse.

There are three degrees of atrioventricular block:

- **1° A-V block** In first-degree A-V block, there is only a delay in atrioventricular conduction of all beats. This is reflected in a prolonged P-R interval in all beats, without any dropped beats (Fig. 15.3).
- **2° A-V block** In second-degree A-V block, there is intermittent dropping of one or more beats. The P wave of the dropped beat is inscribed normally as atrial activation proceeds as usual. Only the QRS complex is missing because of failure of ventricular activation.

  Second-degree A-V block is further classified as Mobitz Type I block and Mobitz Type II block.

  In Mobitz Type I block, there is a gradual lengthening of the P-R interval from beat-to-beat till a P wave is not followed by a QRS complex (Fig. 15.4), indicating a progressively increasing difficulty in A-V nodal transmission. After the dropped beat the P-R interval again shortens, indicating recovery of the A-V node, but then begins to lengthen once again. This sequence of events is referred to as the Wenckebach phenomenon.

  In Mobitz Type II block, the P-R interval remains constant but there is intermittent dropping of beats, with some P waves

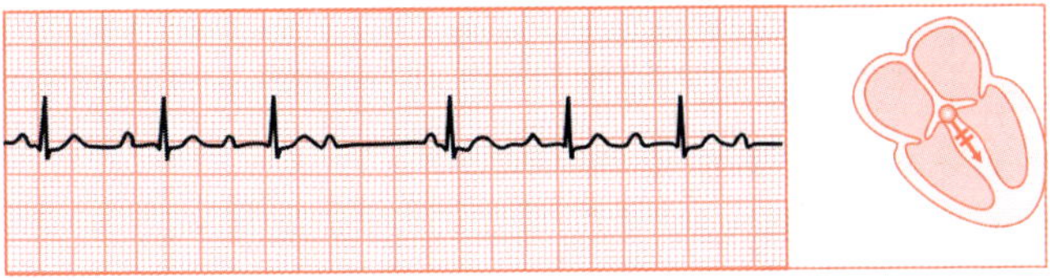

Fig. 15.4: Second-degree A-V block (Mobitz Type I): Wenckebach phenomenon

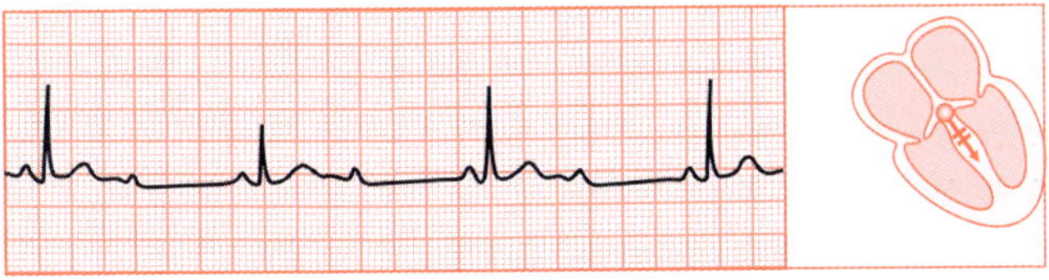

Fig. 15.5: Second-degree A-V block (Mobitz Type II): 2:1 A-V conduction

not followed by a QRS complex (Fig. 15.5). The ratio of the number of P waves to the number of QRS complexes represents the conduction sequence. If every second P wave is blocked, it is 2:1 A-V block and if every third P wave is blocked, it is 3:2 A-V block.

- **3° A-V block** Third-degree A-V block is also known as complete heart block. In this type of A-V block, no sinus beat conducts to the ventricles as all of them get blocked in the A-V node. Therefore, while the atria are activated by the S-A node, the ventricles are activated by a subsidiary pacemaker in the His bundle system or the ventricle.

  In other words, the atria and ventricles work independant of each other and asynchronously, leading to atrioventricular (AV) dissociation.

  In third-degree A-V block, P waves occur at a rate of 60-80 beats/min that represents the discharge rate of the S-A node. The rate of which QRS complexes occur depends upon the location of the subsidiary pacemaker.

If the lower pacemaker is situated in the His bundle system, the ventricular rate is 40-60 beats/min and the QRS complexes are narrow since intraventricular conduction of beats is normal (Fig. 15.6A).

However, if the lower pacemaker is situated in the ventricles, the rate is 20-40 beats/min and the QRS complexes are wide as the ventricles are activated in a slow random fashion (Fig. 15.6B).

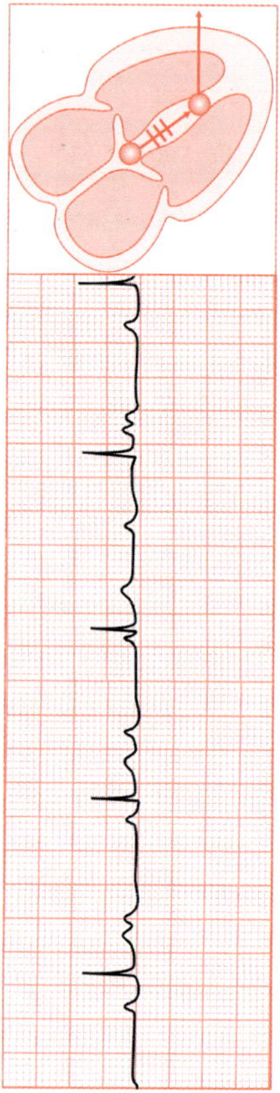

Fig. 15.6A: Third-degree (complete) A-V block: with narrow QRS complexes

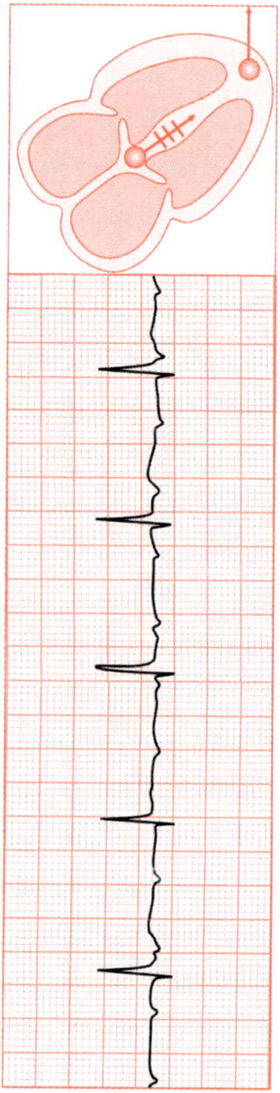

Fig. 15.6B: Third-degree (complete) A-V block: with wide QRS complexes

Clinical Relevance of Pauses

Pause After Premature Beat

The compensatory pause after an atrial premature beat is incomplete while a ventricular premature beat is followed by a complete compensatory pause. This fact helps to differentiate a ventricular premature beat from an atrial premature beat conducted aberrantly to the ventricles.

An inordinately long pause after an atrial premature beat (prolonged sinus node recovery time) indicates sinus node dysfunction, the so called 'sick sinus syndrome'.

The awareness of a ventricular premature beat by the patient and its clinical recognition depend upon the compensatory pause and the increased force of the sinus beat following the premature beat.

Pause After Blocked Premature Beat

Atrial premature beat that fail to conduct to the ventricles produce pauses that resemble those due to S-A block or A-V block. Proper recognition of such pauses is important as their clinical significance and management are different.

Non-conducted atrial premature beats are frequently observed in elderly patients who have advanced A-V nodal disease and in the presence of digitalis toxicity.

Pause Due to Second-Degree S-A Block

Sinoatrial block may be observed in these conditions:

- Drugs, e.g. beta-blockers, diltiazem, digitalis.
- Sinus node dysfunction or sick sinus syndrome.

The "sick sinus syndrome" is a clinical condition caused by a diseased sinus node which fails to produce sufficient impulses. It is observed in elderly patients and is believed to be caused by a degenerative condition (amyloidosis) or infiltration of the atria by a fibrocalcerous process.

- The ECG features of sick sinus syndrome are:

  Sinus bradycardia

  Sinoatrial block

  Slow atrial fibrillation

  Junctional escape rhythm.

- Other clinical features of this syndrome are:

  Inadequate tachycardia with stimuli

  Atropine resistant bradyarrhythmias

  Excessive beta-blocker sensitivity

  Alternating fast and slow rhythms (the "bradytachy" syndrome)

- Symptoms of sick sinus syndrome are:

  Dizziness, syncope or fainting attacks

  Fatigue and dyspnoea from heart failure

  Palpitations and angina pectoris

  Mental confusion and memory defects.

- Treatment of sick sinus syndrome includes:

  Drugs to increase the heart rate, e.g. atropine and sympathomimetic drugs

  Pacemaker insertion if symptoms due to bradycardia are frequent and severe

  Antiarrhythmic drugs for tachyarrhythmias which can be used only if an artificial pacemaker is in place or else they may cause severe bradycardia.

Pause Due to Second-Degree A-V Block

Atrioventricular block (second-degree) may be observed in the following conditions:

- Acute febrile illness

  Rheumatic fever

  Diphtheria

- Drug therapy
  - Digitalis
  - Diltiazem
  - Beta-blockers
- Coronary artery disease
  - Inferior wall infarction
  - Right coronary artery spasm.

The occurrence of A-V block in a febrile illness like rheumatic fever or diphtheria indicates associated myocarditis. The fact that drugs like propranolol and diltiazem can cause A-V block is put to use in the management of atrial tachycardia to reduce the ventricular rate.

Since the A-V node receives its blood supply from the right coronary artery in 90 percent of subjects, transient A-V blocks are observed in inferior wall myocardial infarction caused by occlusion of the right coronary artery. The same may occur when the right coronary artery undergoes spasm.

Mobitz Type I A-V block is often acute in onset, runs a self-limited course, only occasionally produces symptoms, rarely progresses to complete A-V block, carries a good prognosis and often requires no treatment.

Mobitz Type II A-V block is often chronic, almost always pathological, likely to produce symptoms such as dizziness and fainting, may progress to complete A-V block, carries an adverse prognosis and often requires cardiac pacing.

In the management of symptomatic A-V block, although drugs like atropine and adrenalin can temporarily accelerate the ventricular rate, cardiac pacing is the definitive form of treatment especially in patients with recurrent and severe symptoms.

Pauses Causing Bigeminal Rhythm

We have examined above, the various causes of pauses during a regular rhythm. If these pauses occur regularly and are so timed that they follow a pair of beats, they produce a characteristic rhythm called bigeminal rhythm.

The causes of a bigeminal rhythm are:

- Alternate atrial premature beats: (extrasystolic atrial bigeminy)
- Alternate ventricular premature beats (extrasystolic ventricular bigeminy)
- Blocked atrial ectopics after two beats
- 3:2 second-degree sinoatrial block
- 3:2 second-degree atrioventricular block.

CHAPTER 16 Fast Regular Rhythm with Narrow QRS Complexes

REGULAR FAST RHYTHM

A regular cardiac rhythm that exceeds a rate of 100 beats per minute indicates rapid discharge of impulses from the pacemaker governing the rhythm of the heart.

If the QRS complexes during such a rhythm are narrow, it indicates normal intraventricular conduction and that the pacemaker is supraventricular in location, be it the S-A node, the atrial myocardium or the A-V junction.

Let us examine the specific arrhythmias that are associated with these features.

SINUS TACHYCARDIA

The occurrence of sinus node discharge at a rate exceeding 100 beats/min constitutes sinus tachycardia. The rhythm is regular and the P wave as well as QRS morphology are obviously as in normal sinus rhythm (Fig. 16.1).

Sinus tachycardia generally does not exceed a rate of 150 beats/min as the A-V node cannot conduct more than 150 impulses in a minute. Therefore, in sinus tachycardia, the R-R interval ranges from 10 mm (heart rate 150) to 15 mm (heart rate 100).

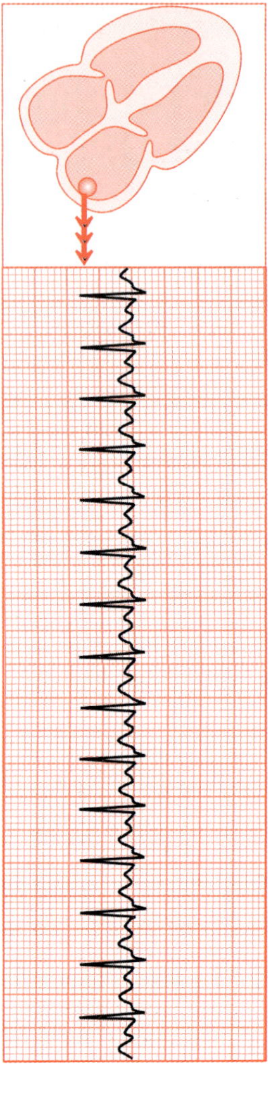

Fig. 16.1: Sinus tachycardia: narrow QRS complexes, rate < 150/min

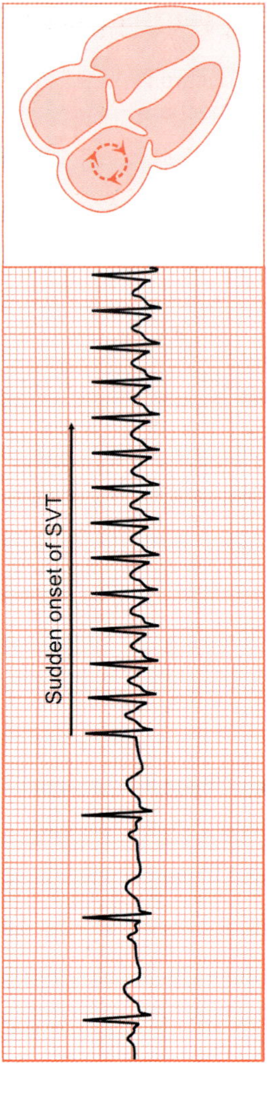

Fig. 16.2: A-V re-entrant tachycardia: narrow QRS complexes, rate > 150/min

ATRIAL TACHYCARDIA

Atrial tachycardia is a fast regular rhythm produced by two possible mechanisms:

- Rapid impulse discharge from ectopic focus in the atrium.
- Repetitive circus movement in a closed re-entrant circuit.

The circuit is either composed of two pathways within the A-V node or consists of an A-V nodal pathway and an accessory bypass tract alongside the A-V node. The two pathways of the re-entrant circuit are connected to each other functionally, to form a closed loop.

An atrial impulse first passes anterogradely down one of the pathways, the other pathway being in the refractory period. The impulse then returns retrogradely through the other pathway which has by now recovered its conductivity. In this way, repetitive circulation of impulses occurs to produce a sustained atrial tachycardia.

The heart rate in paroxysmal atrial tachycardia is 150 to 200 beats per minute (Fig. 16.2) if a re-entrant circuit is involved. It tends to be slower in ectopic atrial tachycardia (120 to 150 beats/min) as the A-V node cannot conduct more than 150 atrial impulses per minute.

The heart rate can exceed a rate of 200 beats/min if a true accessory bypass tract is involved as in the WPW syndrome. This is because in the WPW syndrome, the impulses can bypass the decremental influence of the A-V node by passing down the accessory pathway.

In most cases of atrial tachycardia, the ventricular rate is the same as the atrial rate representing 1:1 A-V conduction. This is always true for a re-entrant tachycardia because the block of even a single impulse can interrupt the continuous reciprocating process and terminate the tachycardia. However, an ectopic atrial tachycardia can coexist with a physiological block such as 2:1 A-V block.

The contour and polarity of the P waves in atrial tachycardia is different from P wave morphology during sinus rhythm. In ectopic atrial tachycardia, the P waves are generally upright while they may be inverted in reciprocating tachycardia, signifying retrograde atrial activation. The P waves are often not discernible in atrial tachycardia as they are fused with the T waves.

The QRS complex of an atrial tachycardia generally has a normal narrow configuration as intraventricular conduction of atrial impulses proceeds as usual. At times, the atrial impulses find one of the two bundle branches refractory to conduction and pass down only one bundle branch. This produces a bundle branch block like configuration of the QRS complexes and is known as aberrant ventricular conduction of an atrial tachycardia.

Other causes of wide QRS complexes during atrial tachycardia are pre-existing conditions producing QRS abnormalities such as true bundle branch block, intraventricular conduction defect or the WPW syndrome.

The differences between sinus tachycardia and atrial tachycardia have been tabulated in Table 16.1.

Table 16.1: Differences between sinus and atrial tachycardia

	Atrial tachycardia	*Sinus tachycardia*
Heart rate	150-220/min	100-150/min
Regularity	Clock-like	Respiratory variation
P wave	Ectopic/Inverted	Normal
Onset	Sudden	Gradual warming up
Effect of vagal maneuvers	Termination	Slowing of rate
ECG during normal rhythm	APCs or WPW syndrome	Often normal

The features of a paroxysmal atrial tachycardia that differentiate it from sinus tachycardia are:

- Heart rate of 150-220 beats/min
- Clock-like regularity of rhythm
- Sudden onset of tachycardia
- P waves different from sinus P waves
- History of recurrent episodes of tachycardia
- Abrupt termination with vagal maneuvers

An atrial tachycardia arising from an ectopic focus can be differentiated from a tachycardia due to a re-entrant mechanism by the features mentioned in Table 16.2.

Table 16.2: Differences between ectopic and re-entrant tachycardia

	Ectopic tachycardia	*Re-entrant tachycardia*
Heart rate	120-150/min	More than 150/min
Onset and offset	Gradual	Sudden
P wave	Ectopic. Visible	Inverted. Rarely visible
A-V block	Can coexist	Never. 1:1 conduction
Effect of vagal meneuvers	Slowing	Termination
Past history	Not significant	Of previous episodes
Organic heart disease	May be present	Generally absent

An atrial tachycardia with aberrant ventricular condition closely resembles a ventricular tachycardia. Features that favour the diagnosis of atrial tachycardia are:

- Clock-like regular rhythm
- Maintained P-QRS relationship
- QRS width less than 0.14 sec
- Stable haemodynamic parameters
- Absence of serious organic heart disease
- Termination with carotid sinus pressure.

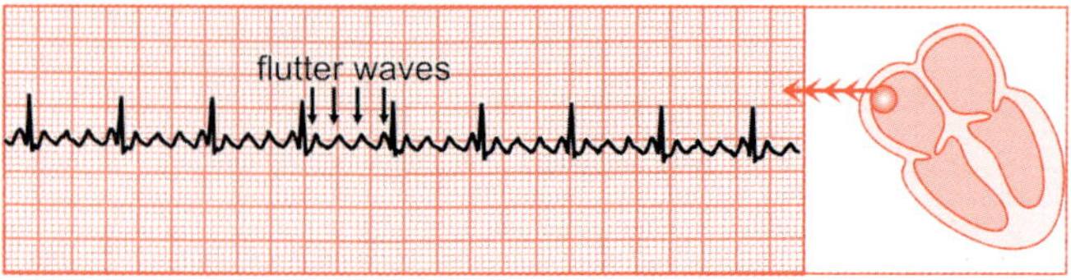

Fig. 16.3: Atrial flutter: discrete F waves, regular ventricular rhythm

ATRIAL FLUTTER

Atrial flutter is a fast rhythm caused by rapid discharge of an ectopic atrial focus or alternatively, a self-perpetuating re-entrant circuit located in the atrium. Therefore, it is obvious that atrial flutter is akin to atrial tachycardia.

The major difference between atrial flutter and atrial tachycardia is in terms of the atrial rate. The atrial rate in atrial flutter is 220-350 beats per minute. The P waves are replaced by flutter waves (F waves) that occur rapidly at this rate and give the base-line a corrugated or saw-toothed appearance (Fig. 16.3).

It is understandable that all flutter waves cannot activate the ventricles. Therefore, there exists a physiological A-V block whereby the ventricular rate is a fraction of the atrial rate. If there is 2:1 physiological A-V block, two flutter waves are followed by one QRS complex while if the block is 4:1, four flutter waves are followed by one QRS complex.

Generally, the even ratios of physiological A-V block (2:1, 4:1) are more common than odd ratios (3:1, 5:1). Assuming an atrial flutter at an atrial rate of 300 beats/min, with 2:1 block, the ventricular rate would be 150 beats/min and with 4:1 block it would be 75 beats/min.

Atrial flutter is quite akin to atrial tachycardia in terms of causation, mechanism and ECG features. The two conditions can be differentiated from each other by the features enumerated in Table 16.3.

Table 16.3: Differences between atrial flutter and atrial tachycardia

	Atrial flutter	*Atrial tachycardia*
Atrial rate	220-350/min	150-220/min
Ventricular rate	1/2 or 1/4 of atrial rate (2:1 or 4:1 A-V block)	Same as atrial rate (1:1 A-V conduction)
P waves	Saw-tooth like flutter waves	Ectopic/inverted P waves
Effect of carotid sinus pressure	Increased degree of A-V block	Termination in PAT. Slowing in ectopic tachycardia

Atrial flutter with 2:1 physiological A-V block resembles a sinus tachycardia at a rate of 120-150 beats/min if one of the two flutter waves is buried in the QRS complex and the other is mistaken for the P wave. The diagnosis of atrial flutter can be clinched if after carotid sinus pressure, the degree of A-V block increases and both the flutter waves become evident.

Clinical Relevance of a Fast Regular Narrow-QRS Rhythm

Sinus Tachycardia

Sinus tachycardia represents response of the S-A node to a variety of physiological and pathological stimuli, mediated by the nervous and hormonal control over the pacemaker discharge rate.

The causes of sinus tachycardia are:

- Exercise and emotion
- Fever and volume depletion
- Hypoxemia and anaemia
- Hypotension and heart failure
- Thyrotoxicosis and myocarditis
- Caffeine, nicotine and alcohol
- Atropine and sympathomimetics

In febrile patients, for each degree Fahrenheit rise in temperature, the heart rate rises by 8 to 10 beats/min. A sinus tachycardia in excess of the predicted rate is a feature of myocarditis, rheumatic fever or bacterial endocarditis.

A sinus tachycardia at a rate less than expected in a febrile person is known as relative bradycardia and is observed in typhoid fever and in brucellosis.

Failure to develop sinus tachycardia in reponse to a physiological or pathological stimulus and in the absence of beta-blocker or calcium-blocker therapy is a sign of sinus node dysfunction, the so called sick sinus syndrome.

Sinus tachycardia is not a primary arrhythmia and therefore, treatment should be directed towards the basic underlying condition. Examples are antipyretics for fever, oxygen for hypoxemia, fluids for volume depletion and tranquilizers for emotional upset.

Specific therapy should be instituted when sinus tachycardia is an expression of the underlying disease. Such diseases include severe anaemia, thyrotoxicosis, congestive heart failure, rheumatic fever and bacterial endocarditis.

Withdrawal of smoking, beverages, spices, anticholinergic drugs and adrenergic agents is mandatory to control the tachycardia. Propranolol and mild tranquilizers are indicated for supportive therapy of sinus tachycardia associated with anxiety, anaemia and thyrotoxicosis

Atrial Tachycardia

As a series of three or more successive atrial ectopic beats constitutes an atrial tachycardia, the causes of ectopic atrial tachycardia are similar to those of atrial premature beats. These include:

- Rheumatic fever
- Digitalis toxicity
- Thyrotoxicosis

- Myocarditis
- Adrenergic drugs
- Cardiac surgery

Paroxysmal re-entrant atrial tachycardia is most often based on a reciprocal mechanism involving a bypass tract or dual intra-nodal pathway. Episodes of atrial tachycardia are one of the manifestation of pre-excitation syndrome, the WPW syndrome.

In the absence of WPW syndrome, paroxysmal atrial tachycardia (PAT) is generally not associated with organic heart disease. If properly managed, PAT does not alter life-expectancy and has an excellent prognosis.

PAT coexisting with the WPW syndrome carries a poorer prognosis because of the risk of degeneration into ventricular tachycardia.

A re-entrant atrial tachycardia always exists with 1:1 A-V conduction since the reciprocating circuit would break with the block of even a single beat. This is also the reason why vagal stimulation methods and drugs that block the A-V node can terminate the tachycardia.

On the other hand, an ectopic atrial tachycardia can coexist with A-V block and is popularly known as 'PAT with block'. Digitalis toxicity is the most common cause of this rhythm.

Symptoms due to atrial tachycardia depend upon the atrial rate, the duration of the tachycardia and the presence of heart disease.

A fast atrial tachycardia causes palpitation and neck pulsations. Angina pectoris may occur due to increased myocardial oxygen demand and reduced coronary filling time.

Prolonged atrial tachycardia can cause dizziness or syncope due to decline in cardiac output secondary to a shortened ventricular filling time and loss of atrial contribution to ventricular filling.

Atrial tachycardia needs to be differentiated clinically and electrocardiographically from various other rhythms that closely simulate it.

Differentiation from sinus tachycardia is important since atrial tachycardia needs more aggressive treatment.

The causation and to some extent, the response to treatment of ectopic atrial tachycardia is somewhat different from that of re-entrant tachycardia and the two need to be differentiated electrocardiographically.

Finally, atrial tachycardia with aberrant ventricular conduction needs to be identified as distinct from ventricular tachycardia since their causation, clinical presentation, prognosis and treatment are entirely different.

The Wolff-Parkinson-White (WPW) syndrome is a distinct electrocardiographic entity wherein an accessory pathway, the Bundle of Kent, connects the atrial to the ventricular myocardium, bypassing the A-V node. This produces abnormalities of the QRS complex, P-R interval, S-T segment and the T wave, during sinus rhythm.

The clinical importance of the WPW syndrome lies in the fact that it predisposes to paroxysmal atrial tachycardia since the bypass tract forms a re-entrant circuit with the regular conduction pathway. Paroxysmal tachycardia in the presence of WPW syndrome needs to be differentiated from a PAT without the accessory pathway since its management is somewhat different.

A paroxysm of atrial tachycardia in the presence of an underlying WPW syndrome is suggested if it meets one of the following criteria:

- ECG recorded in sinus rhythm shows a short P-R interval, delta wave and a wide QRS complex.
- The ventricular rate exceeds 200 beats/min indicating absence of physiological A-V block.
- Inverted P waves are observed indicating retrograde atrial activation and conduction.

There are several modalities of treatment of PAT. Since reentry through an intra-nodal pathway or a bypass tract accounts for 90 percent of PAT, we shall first discuss the management of re-entrant PAT.

The first step is to try methods of vagal stimulation so as to reduce A-V conduction and consequently the ventricular rate. Vagal maneuvers that may be attempted include carotid sinus massage, supraorbital pressure, Valsalva maneuver or immersion of face in ice-cold water.

If vagal maneuvers fail to abort the tachycardia, a drug acting on the A-V node may be given intravenously.

The protocol of drug therapy for PAT is:

Adenosine 6 mg IV over 1-3 sec.; repeat 12 mg IV after 1-2 min.; repeat 12 mg IV after another 1-2 min; till sinus rhythm is restored or 30 mg is given.

OR

Diltiazem 15-20 mg (0.25 mg/kg) IV over 2 min; repeat 20-25 mg (0.35 mg/kg) IV over 2 min after 15 min if needed.

OR

Amiodarone 150 mg IV over 10 min (15 mg/min); repeat 150 mg IV over 10 min; repeat every 10 min if needed.

Oral diltiazem, amiodarone or metoprolol is prescribed after restoration of sinus rhythm to prevent recurrence of PAT.

In drug-refractory atrial tachycardia, delivering a single programmed extrastimulus by atrial pacing can break the re-entrant circuit and restore sinus rhythm.

Electrical cardioversion with 100-200 Joules is the treatment of choice for atrial tachycardia with deranged haemodynamics and low cardiac output.

Surgical ablation of the A-V junction may be considered as a last resort in frequent, recurrent drug-refractory PAT which however, makes the concomitant insertion of a permanent pacemaker mandatory.

The management of ectopic atrial tachycardia is similar to that of PAT with these differences:

- vagal maneuvers are less likely to be effective
- digoxin is to be avoided as it causes ectopic beats

- programmed extra-stimulus cannot restore sinus rhythm
- long-term prophylactic treatment is not indicated
- electrical cardioversion and surgical ablation have no role.

The management of paroxysmal atrial tachycardia in the presence of WPW syndrome is also somewhat different.

- vagal maneuvers would be useful only if anterograde conduction occurs through the A-V node.
- digitalis is contraindicated as it enhances conduction down the accessory pathway and may precipitate ventricular fibrillation.
- diltiazem and metoprolol reduce tolerance to the high ventricular rate and precipitate congestive heart failure.
- Class I antiarrhythmic drugs like procainamide may be useful as they prolong the refractory period of atrial myocardium and the accessory pathway.
- amiodarone is the antiarrhythmic agent of choice for the long-term treatment and prevention of arrhythmias associated with the WPW syndrome.

Urgent electrical cardioversion is life-saving in atrial tachycardia associated with unstable haemodynamic parameters.

The availability of sophisticated electrophysiological studies to identify and locate a bypass tract and the development of laser-assisted surgery have revolutionalized the management of WPW syndrome.

Radiofrequency ablation (RFA) of the bypass tract can be offered to patients who report recurrent and frequent symptomatic episodes of PAT that produce haemodynamic compromise and are refractory to drug therapy.

Cardioversion should be preceded by intravenous heparin and a transoesophageal ECHO to exclude an atrial clot. It should be followed up by oral anticoagulation for 4 weeks.

Atrial Flutter

Atrial flutter is quite akin to ectopic tachycardia electrocardiographically, differing from it only in terms of the atrial rate. In terms of causation too, atrial flutter closely resembles atrial tachycardia.

Common causes are:

- Rheumatic heart disease
- Acute respiratory failure
- Thyrotoxicosis
- Myocarditis
- Pericarditis
- Cardiac surgery

Compared to its better known counterpart called atrial fibrillation, atrial flutter is less common and generally short-lived. It causes fewer symptoms and is less likely to cause a left atrial thrombus and subsequent risk of systemic embolization.

As far as the management of atrial flutter is concerned, the heart rate may be controlled by diltiazem or metoprolol as in atrial tachycardia. If conversion to sinus rhythm or to atrial fibrillation is the goal, digoxin or amiodarone may be used.

Digoxin converts atrial flutter to fibrillation with an increase in atrial rate. However, this is of advantage since the ventricular rate declines as the degree of concealed conduction increases. When digitalis is stopped, this often restores sinus thythm.

If the patient's clinical status is unsatisfactory with angina, hypotension or heart failure, electrical cardioversion with a low energy shock of 10 to 50 Joules is the most effective form of treatment. In fact, atrial flutter is the most responsive of the tachyarrhythmias that revert with electrical cardioversion.

CHAPTER 17

Normal Regular Rhythm with Narrow QRS Complexes

REGULAR NORMAL RHYTHM

A regular cardiac rhythm at a rate of 60 to 100 beats per minute is considered to be a normal rhythm.

If the QRS complexes during such a rhythm are narrow, it indicates normal intraventricular conduction and that the pacemaker is supraventricular in location. The pacemaker may be the S-A node, in the atrial myocardium or at the A-V junction.

Let us examine the specific arrhythmias that are associated with these features.

NORMAL SINUS RHYTHM

The occurrence of sinus node discharge at a rate of 60 to 100 beats/min constitutes a normal sinus rhythm.

The rhythm is regular, the P wave and QRS complex are normal in morphology and they are related to each other with a 1:1 relationship.

ATRIAL TACHYCARDIA WITH 2:1 A-V BLOCK

In atrial tachycardia, the atrial rate varies from 150 to 200 beats/min. If all atrial impulses are conducted to the ventricles, the ventricular rate is identical.

If however, there exists a physiological 2:1 A-V block and every alternate P wave is followed by a QRS complex, the ventricular rate is half of the atrial rate or 75 to 100 beats/min.

Such as rhythm superficially resembles a normal sinus rhythm with the difference that the P-P interval between successive P waves reflects an atrial rate of 150 to 200 beats/min.

ATRIAL FLUTTER WITH 4:1 A-V BLOCK

In atrial flutter the atrial rate varies from 220 to 350 beats/min. Since all atrial impulses cannot conduct to the ventricles at this rate, there exists a physiological A-V block and the ventricular rate is a fraction of the atrial rate.

If the physiological block is 4: 1 and every fourth flutter wave is followed by QRS complex the ventricular rate is one-fourth of the atrial rate or 60 to 80 beats/min.

Such a rhythm superficially resembles a normal sinus rhythm with the difference that the P waves are replaced by rapidly occurring flutter waves.

Atrial flutter can be differentiated from atrial tachycardia (atrial rate 150 to 200 beats/min) with 2:1 block by the fact that the F-F interval between successive F waves indicates an atrial rate of 220 to 350 beats/min.

JUNCTIONAL TACHYCARDIA

Junctional tachycardia is an ectopic rhythm originating from a latent subsidiary pacemaker located in the A-V junction. Normally, this pacemaker is subdued when the cardiac rhythm is governed by the S-A node. However, when the junctional pacemaker undergoes enhancement of its inherent automaticity, it produces a junctional tachycardia.

This rhythm is also known as non-paroxysmal junctional tachycardia to differentiate it from extrasystolic junctional tachycardia produced by a series of three or more junctional premature beats. Non-paroxysmal junctional tachycardia is also known as accelerated junctional rhythm.

Junctional tachycardia produces a regular rhythm at a rate of 60 to 100 beats/min which is greater than the inherent rate of the junctional pacemaker (40 to 60 beats/min). The QRS complexes are narrow as in normal sinus rhythm (Fig. 17.1).

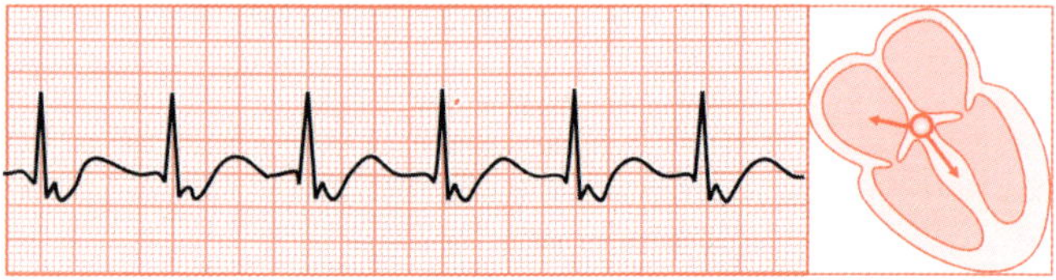

Fig. 17.1: Accelerated junctional rhythm: inverted P waves just follow the QRS complexes

The distinctive feature of a junctional tachycardia is the typical relationship between P waves and QRS complexes. If the atria are activated retrogradely from the junctional pacemaker, the P waves are inverted and related to the QRS complexes. They may just precede, just follow or be buried in the QRS complexes because of near-simultaneous atrial and ventricular activation.

If the atria continue to be activated by the S-A node, the P waves are upright and unrelated to the QRS complexes. In that case, the junctional pacemaker only activates the ventricles. The ventricular rate is then slightly greater than the atrial rate, that is, the R-R interval is slightly shorter than the P-P interval.

Consequently, there is a progressive shortening of the P-R interval in successive beats till the P wave merges in the QRS complex and then follows it. The P wave, so to say, marches through the QRS complex. This form of atrioventricular dissociation is called isorhythmic A-V dissociation since atrial and ventricular rates are nearly similar.

The P-QRS relationship mentioned above is typical of a rhythm originating from the AV junctional pacemaker. Inverted P waves just precede, just follow or are buried in the QRS complexes.

A junctional escape rhythm has similar features but occurs at a slower rate of 40 to 60 beats/min which is the inherent rate of the junctional pacemaker.

An extrasystolic junctional tachycardia can be differentiated from accelerated junctional rhythm by the fact that it starts abruptly, is often paroxysmal in nature and the ventricular rate exceeds 120 beats/min. The two conditions can be differentiated by features mentioned in Table 17.1.

Table 17.1: Junctional tachycardia versus junctional rhythm

	Extrasystolic junctional tachycardia	*Accelerated junctional rhythm*
Onset	Abrupt	Slow warm-up
Occurrence	Paroxysmal	Sustained
Ventricular rate	120-150/min	60-100/min

Clinical Relevance of a Normal Regular Narrow-QRS Rhythm

Normal Sinus Rhythm

A rhythm originating from the S-A node at a rate of 60 to 100 beats/min is a normal sinus cardiac rhythm. It is the most common, but by no means the only cause of a rhythm at this rate.

Atrial Tachycardia with Fixed A-V Block

A fast atrial rhythm such as atrial tachycardia or atrial flutter, when associated with a fixed degree of physiological A-V block, can also produce a normal ventricular rhythm at 60 to 100 beats/min.

Junctional Tachycardia

A junctional tachycardia due to enhanced automaticity of the junctional pacemaker may be observed in:

- Digitalis toxicity
- Rheumatic carditis
- Inferior wall infarction
- Cardiac surgery
- Thyrotoxicosis.

When a febrile child develops a junctional tachycardia, rheumatic fever with carditis should be suspected. Thyrotoxicosis is a frequent cause of various atrial tachyarrhythmias including junctional tachycardia.

In a coronary care unit, junctional tachycardia is often observed in cases of inferior wall myocardial infarction after they have recovered from A-V block.

Open heart surgery especially septal repair around the A-V node, may be a cause of junctional tachycardia in the postoperative period.

If a patient is on digitalis for atrial fibrillation, regularization of the cardiac rhythm, even if sinus rhythm is not restored, is often due to the onset of junctional tachycardia. This constitutes one of the markers of digitalis toxicity.

It is difficult and often futile to differentiate an extrasystolic junctional tachycardia from an ectopic tachycardia of atrial origin. They are both supraventricular tachycardias and similar in aetiology, significance and management.

Junctional tachycardia is generally asymptomatic as it occurs at the same rate-range as sinus rhythm. Moreover, its onset does not cause significant clinical deterioration as ventricular activation is normal. Only the loss of atrial contribution to ventricular filling (A-V dissociation), can cause slight decline in cardiac output.

Active treatment of junctional tachycardia is generally not required as it is asymptomatic and has few haemodynamic consequences.

If treatment is required as in patients with poor cardiac reserve, management of the precipitating event is the first goal. This includes management of digitalis intoxication, treatment of rheumatic carditis and control of thyrotoxicosis.

If these do not suffice, atropine can be given to accelerate the sinus rate, overdrive the junctional rhythm and eliminate atrioventricular dissociation.

Antiarrhythmic drugs, electrical cardioversion and external pacing are unnecessary while vagal stimulation methods have no role in the management of junctional tachycardia.

18 CHAPTER

Fast Irregular Rhythm with Narrow QRS Complexes

IRREGULAR FAST RHYTHM

A cardiac rhythm that exceeds a rate of 100 beats per minute indicates rapid discharge of impulses from the pacemaker governing the rhythm of the heart.

If the QRS complexes during such a rhythm are narrow, it indicates normal intraventricular conduction and that the pacemaker is supraventricular in location.

Further, if the rhythm is irregular, it signifies a variability either in impulse origin or in impulse conduction through the A-V node.

Let us examine the specific arrhythmias that are associated with these features.

ATRIAL TACHYCARDIA WITH VARYING A-V BLOCK

In atrial tachycardia, the atrial rate varies from 150 to 220 beats/min. If all atrial impulses are conducted to the ventricles, the ventricular rate is identical.

However, if some atrial impulses are blocked in the A-V node and this physiological A-V block is variable, the QRS complexes occur at varying intervals to produce an irregular rhythm.

ATRIAL FLUTTER WITH VARYING A-V BLOCK

In atrial flutter, the atrial rate varies from 220 to 350 beats/min. Since all atrial impulses cannot conduct to the ventricles at this rate, there exists a physiological A-V block and the ventricular rate is a fraction of the atrial rate.

Generally, the degree of A-V block is fixed and occurs in even ratios such as 2:1, 4:1 and 8:1. If this physiological A-V block is variable, the QRS complexes occur at varying intervals to produce an irregular rhythm.

MULTIFOCAL ATRIAL TACHYCARDIA

Ectopic atrial tachycardia is a fast rhythm produced by a rapid discharge of impulses from a single ectopic atrial focus. If impulses arise from numerous atrial foci, it constitutes a multifocal atrial tachycardia or a chaotic atrial rhythm.

Multifocal atrial tachycardia is a fast rhythm at a rate of 100 to 150 beats/min characterized by a beat-to-beat variability in P wave configuration representing a changing focus of origin of impulses (Fig. 18.1).

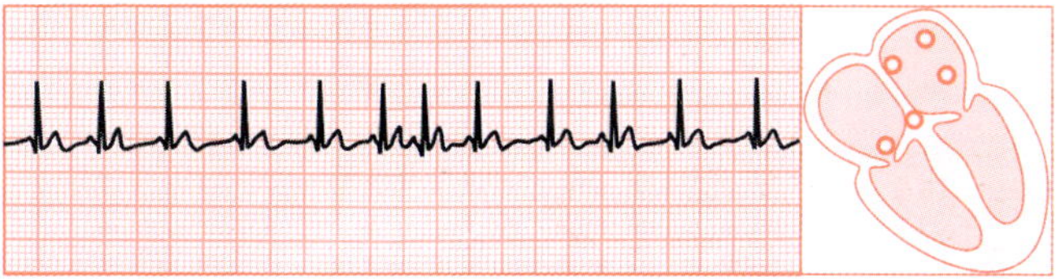

Fig. 18.1: Multifocal atrial tachycardia: different P wave configurations

It may not be possible to select the dominant P wave of sinus origin. The P-R interval is also variable because of variability in A-V conduction time, depending upon the focus of origin. Some P waves are premature, others are blocked and they vary in morphology from being upright to inverted.

The ventricular rhythm is irregular because of the varying degree of prematurity of atrial impulses and the occurrence of blocked atrial beats.

Multifocal atrial tachycardia needs to be differentiated from multiple atrial premature beats occurring frequently during sinus rhythm. In the latter case, it is possible to select the dominant P waves of sinus origin. Moreover, the abnormal P waves occur prematurely and the QRS complexes that succeed them are followed by compensatory pauses.

Multifocal atrial tachycardia (MAT) also closely resembles atrial fibrillation, since the ventricular rate is irregular in both rhythms. However, definite P waves are discernible in MAT while they are absent or replaced by fibrillatory waves (f waves) in atrial fibrillation.

ATRIAL FIBRILLATION

Atrial fibrillation is a grossly irregular fast rhythm produced by the functional fractionation of the atria into numerous tissue islets. Therefore, instead of the sinus impulse spreading evenly and contiguously to all parts of atria, these islets are in various stages of excitation and recovery. Consequently, atrial activation is chaotic and ineffectual in causing haemodynamic pumping.

Although 400 to 500 fibrillatory impulses reach the A-V node per minute, only 100 to 160 of them succeed in eliciting a ventricular response while others are blocked due to A-V nodal refractoriness. The random activation of the ventricles produces a grossly irregular ventricular rhythm.

The hallmark of atrial fibrillation is absence of discrete P waves. Instead, there are numerous, small, irregular fibrillatory waves (f waves) that are difficult to identify individually but produce a ragged base-line (Fig. 18.2).

In longstanding atrial fibrillation, these undulations are minimal and produce a nearly flat base-line. As mentioned earlier, the

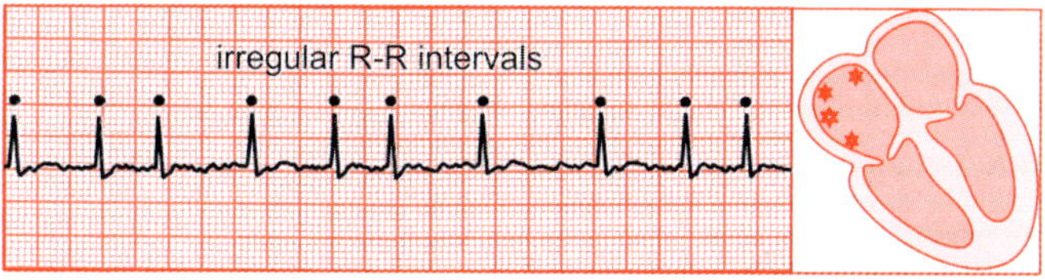

Fig. 18.2: Atrial fibrillation: fine f waves, irregular rhythm

ventricular rate is grossly irregular and varies from 100 to 160 beats per minute.

Atrial fibrillation can be differentiated from multifocal atrial tachycardia (MAT) by the fact that P waves are absent or replaced by fibrillatory waves while definite P waves are discernible in MAT.

Atrial fibrillation can be differentiated from atrial flutter by the following features:

- absence of P waves
- irregular ventricular rate

At times, precise differentiation between the two may be difficult and the rhythm is then known as "flutter-fibrillation", "coarse fibrillation" or "impure flutter". The differences between atrial flutter and atrial fibrillation are enlisted in Table 18.1.

Table 18.1: Differences between atrial flutter and atrial fibrillation

	Atrial flutter	*Atrial fibrillation*
Atrial rate	220-350 beats/min	Over 350 beats/min
Ventricular rate	Regular. Half to one-fourth of atrial rate	Variable. No relation to atrial rate
Atrial activity	Visible flutter (F) waves Saw-toothed base-line	Fine fibrillatory (f) waves Ragged base-line
Ventricular activity	Constant R-R interval	Variable R-R interval

Clinical Relevance of a Fast Irregular Narrow-QRS Rhythm

Atrial Tachycardia with Varying A-V Block

The occurrence of a fast rhythm such as atrial tachycardia or atrial flutter with a variable interval between QRS complexes indicates a variability in conduction of the atrial impulses through the AV node.

Only an ectopic atrial tachycardia and not re-entrant atrial tachycardia can coexist with A-V block. 'PAT with block' is a popular term for this condition and digitalis toxicity is the most common cause of this rhythm.

Multifocal Atrial Tachycardia

The most frequent cause (in 80 to 90% cases) of multifocal atrial tachycardia is chronic obstructive lung disease with corpulmonale and respiratory failure in a seriously ill elderly patient.

Aggravating factors that often coexist are:

- Respiratory tract infection
- Theophylline or digitalis
- Coronary artery disease
- Hypoxia and hypercapnia
- Electrolyte imbalance.

Multifocal atrial tachycardia not only mimics but often heralds the onset of atrial fibrillation. It has serious prognostic implications and carries a high mortality rate.

The treatment of aggravating factors and improvement of the pulmonary condition are the most important principles in the management of multifocal atrial tachycardia.

Necessary measures include treatment of infection with antibiotics, withdrawal of offending drugs, correcting electrolyte imbalance and administering oxygen.

Multifocal atrial tachycardia is not only refractory to antiarrhythmic drugs like verapamil, beta-blockers and digitalis but these can worsen the cardio-respiratory status and are hence to be avoided.

Atrial Fibrillation

Atrial fibrillation may be observed in virtually all forms of organic heart disease. Causes of atrial fibrillation are:

- Persistent atrial fibrillation

  Congenital heart disease (ASD)

  Rheumatic heart disease (MS)

  Coronary artery disease (MR)

  Hypertensive heart disease

  Ideopathic cardiomyopathy

  Constrictive pericarditis

  Cardiac trauma or surgery.

- Paroxysmal atrial fibrillation

  Acute alcoholic intoxication

  Recurrent pulmonary embolism

  Thyrotoxicosis

  WPW syndrome

  Lone atrial fibrillation.

In atrial fibrillation, the ventricular rate generally varies from 100 to 150 beats per minute. Faster rates are observed in children, patients of thyrotoxicosis and in the presence of WPW syndrome.

Slower rates are observed during drug treatment with propranolol/ atenolol or verapamil/diltiazem as these drugs block the A-V node. Elderly patients with A-V nodal disease may also manifest slow atrial fibrillation.

Regularization of the ventricular rate in a patient on digitalis for atrial fibrillation indicates the onset of junctional tachycardia and is a manifestation of digitalis toxicity.

Symptoms due to atrial fibrillation depend upon:

- The ventricular rate
- The severity of heart disease
- The effectiveness of treatment

The symptoms frequently observed in atrial fibrillation along with their causation are:

- Palpitations (fast heart rate)
- Angina (increased myocardial oxygen demand and shortened coronary filling time)
- Fatigue (low cardiac output due to loss of atrial contribution to ventricular filling)
- Dyspnoea (pulmonary congestion due to ineffectual atrial contraction)
- Regional ischemia (systemic embolization from atrial thrombus).

Atrial fibrillation may be life-threatening in these situations:

- Low cardiac output state with pulmonary edema due to left ventricular dysfunction.
- Non-compliant ventricle when atrial contribution to ventricular filling is crucial.
- WPW syndrome where conduction of impulses down the accessory pathway can precipitate ventricular tachycardia or fibrillation.
- Injudicious treatment of atrial fibrillation such as digitalis usage in WPW syndrome and diltiazem or propranolol for sick sinus syndrome.

Clinical signs of atrial fibrillation are:

- *Pulse* Irregular and fast pulse rate; pulse deficit which is radial pulse rate less than the heart rate counted by cardiac auscultation.

- *BP* Low systolic blood pressure; variable pulse pressure
- *JVP* Raised jugular venous pressure; absent 'a' waves
- *Heart sounds* of the first heart sound. Beat-to-beat variability in the intensity.

Various modalities of treatment are available for the management of atrial fibrillation, the judicious use of which can result in clinical improvement of most patients.

- *Anti-arrhythmic drugs* If haemodynamics of the patient are stable, it suffices to control the ventricular rate by a drug that prolongs the refractory period of the A-V node.

  Diltiazem or amiodarone may be administered intravenously to hasten control of heart rate. Doses of these drugs are:

  Diltiazem 15-20 mg over 2 min; repeat after 15 min.

  Amiodarone 150 mg over 10 min; repeat after 10 min.

  Oral diltiazem, amiodarone or metoprolol can be prescribed for long-term administration but should be avoided in the presence of heart failure in which case digoxin is preferable.

  These drugs are contraindicated in the presence of WPW syndrome where A-V nodal block would increase the conduction of impulses down the accessory pathway and hence, the likelihood of ventricular tachycardia.

  Amiodarone is very effective in the prevention of paroxysmal atrial fibrillation. Moreover, it is effective and safe in the presence of the WPW syndrome as it suppresses conduction of impulses down the accessory pathway.

- *Anti-coagulants* Long-standing atrial fibrillation produces stasis of blood in the left atrium and promotes the development of thrombi in the atrial cavity and atrial appendage.

  Dislodged fragments of these thrombi can enter the systemic circulation as emboli and settle down in any arterial territory to produce effects of regional ischemia.

Examples are blindness due to retinal artery occlusion, hemiparesis due to cerebral circulation impairment and ischemia of a limb due to brachioradial or ileofemoral obstruction.

Anti-coagulants such as caumarin and warfarin are required for long-term use in chronic atrial fibrillation to reduce likelihood of systemic embolization. This particularly applies to patients of rheumatic heart disease and prosthetic valve recepients as well as those with previous history of thromboembolism.

Anti-coagulation is also indicated two weeks before and several weeks after electrical cardioversion since restoration of sinus rhythm and atrial function is likely to expel systemic emboli.

- *Electrical cardioversion* If the patient's clinical status is poor and hemodynamics are unstable, electrical cardioversion with 100 to 200 Joules energy is the treatment of choice in an attempt to restore sinus rhythm.

  There are two requisites before cardioversion is attempted. Firstly, the patient should not have received digitalis in the previous 48 hours. Secondly, anti-coagulation should be initiated before cardioversion and continued for atleast 4 weeks later since atrial thrombi are likely to dislodge as emboli, once sinus rhythm is restored.

  It is difficult to restore sinus rhythm with cardioversion if atrial fibrillation is of more than one year duration and the left atrium is enlarged beyond 4.5 cm in diameter.

- *A-V nodal ablation* When all conventional remedies have been exhausted and a number of investigational agents have failed to treat atrial fibrillation, a final option is to ablate the A-V node or an accessory pathway, if it exists.

  This can be performed as radiofrequency ablation (RFA) or laser-assisted surgery. However, this is a major step and suitable only for a minority of cases as life is then dependent upon a permanent ventricular pacemaker.

19 CHAPTER

Fast Regular Rhythm with Wide QRS Complexes

FAST WIDE-QRS RHYTHM

A regular cardiac rhythm that exceeds a rate of 100 beats per minute indicates rapid discharge of impulses from the pacemaker governing the rhythm of the heart.

If the QRS complexes during such a rhythm are wide, three possibilities have to be considered.

- The rhythm is ventricular in origin in which case ventricular activation is through myocardium and not the specialized conduction system
- The rhythm is supraventricular in origin but impulses are conducted aberrantly to the ventricles through one of the two branches of the His bundle
- The rhythm is supraventricular in origin but there are preexisting wide QRS complexes

Let us go into the individual features of these rhythms.

VENTRICULAR TACHYCARDIA

Ventricular tachycardia is a fast regular rhythm produced by two possible mechanisms:

- Enhanced automaticity of a latent ventricular pacemaker producing rapid discharge of impulses.

- Repetitive circus movement of an impulse in a closed re-entrant circuit around a fixed anatomical substrate in the ventricular myocardium.

The heart rate in ventricular tachycardia is generally 150 to 200 beats per minute. The rhythm is usually slightly irregular in contrast to the perfect regularity of an atrial tachycardia.

The QRS complexes are bizarre and wide, exceeding 0.14 sec in width and do not conform to a bundle branch block pattern (Fig. 19.1).

The atria may continue to be activated by the S-A node but the P-waves are generally not visible as they are buried in the wide QRS complexes.

During ventricular tachycardia, the QRS pattern in all precordial leads is similar (concordant pattern) and the R/S ratio in lead V_6 is less than 1. Moreover, there is a leftward deviation of the mean QRS axis.

A ventricular tachycardia closely resembles an atrial tachycardia that is conducted aberrantly to the ventricles. Features that favour the diagnosis of ventricular tachycardia are:

- Slight irregularity of rhythm
- Lack of P-QRS relationship
- QRS width > 0.14 sec with bizarre shape
- Compromised hemodynamic parameters
- Presence of serious organic heart disease
- No response to carotid sinus pressure.

A particular type of ventricular tachycardia called polymorphic ventricular tachycardia is characterized by beat-to-beat variation of the QRS complex amplitude and direction (Fig. 19.2).

Since this gives the appearance of rotation of QRS complexes around the isoelectric line, it is designated as Torsade de pointes which literally means 'torsion of points".

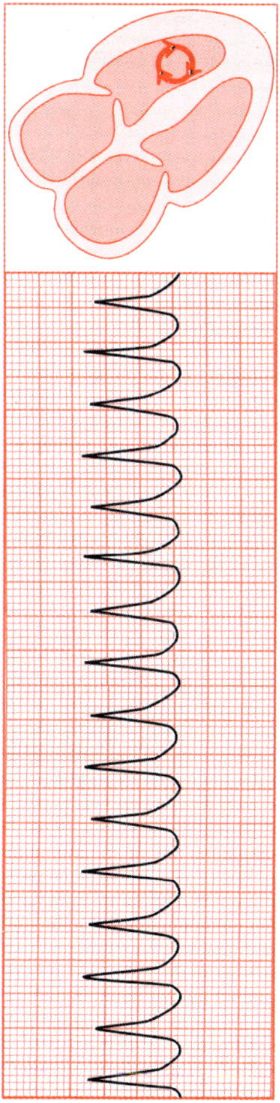

Fig. 19.1: Ventricular tachycardia: wide monomorphic QRS complexes

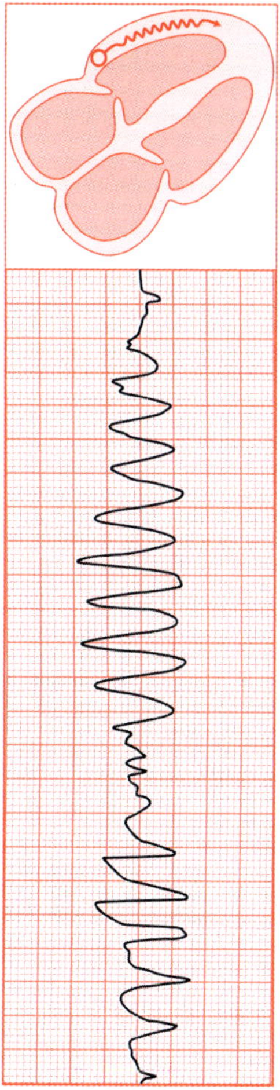

Fig. 19.2: Polymorphic ventricular tachycardia: changing QRS configuration

Torsade de pointes is, as a rule, associated with prolongation of the Q-T interval. The prolonged Q-T interval favours the occurrence of a ventricular premature beat that coincides with the T-wave of the preceding beat (R-on-T phenomenon) and initiates the ventricular tachycardia.

SUPRAVENTRICULAR TACHYCARDIA WITH ABERRANT VENTRICULAR CONDUCTION

Most often, a supraventricular tachycardia is characterized by narrow QRS complexes as a result of synchronized ventricular activation through the specialized conduction system.

Occasionally, the supraventricular impulses find one of the two bundle branches refractory to conduction. In that case, the impulses are conducted only through the other bundle branch producing a situation of aberrant ventricular conduction. Understandably, the QRS complexes conform to a bundle branch block pattern.

The differences between ventricular tachycardia and supraventricular tachycardia with aberrant ventricular conduction are given in Table 19.1.

Table 19.1: Differences between ventricular tachycardia and SVT with aberrant conduction

	Ventricular tachycardia	*SVT with aberrancy*
Regularity of rhythm	Slightly irregular	Clock-like regularity
P-QRS relationship	P waves not seen	P waves may be seen
	Unrelated	Related
QRS width and morphology	>0.14 sec. Bizarre	0.12-0.14 sec. Triphasic
Pattern in V_1 to V_6	rS in V_1 to V_6	RsR' in V_1 Rs in V_6
QRS in lead V_6	rS R<S	Rs R>S
QRS axis	Leftward	Normal
Haemodynamics	Compromised	Stable
Organic heart disease	Often present	Often absent
Response to carotid sinus pressure	No response	Slowing or termination

SUPRAVENTRICULAR TACHYCARDIA WITH PRE-EXISTING QRS ABNORMALITY

It is known that certain conditions produce an abnormality of ventricular conduction even in normal sinus rhythm, causing an abnormality of QRS morphology.

Three well known examples are:

- Bundle branch block
- WPW syndrome
- Intraventricular conduction defect

If a supraventricular tachycardia occurs in the presence of a pre-existing QRS abnormality, it is naturally expected to have wide QRS complexes.

A bundle branch block produces a triphasic QRS contour while an intraventricular conduction defect results in bizarre QRS morphology. The WPW syndrome is characterized by a delta wave on the ascending limb of the QRS complex.

Clinical Relevance of a Fast Regular Wide–QRS Rhythm

Ventricular Tachycardia

A series of three or more successive ventricular ectopic beats constitutes a ventricular tachycardia.

A ventricular tachycardia that lasts for more than 30 seconds and requires cardioversion for termination is called sustained ventricular tachycardia. A non-sustained ventricular tachycardia lasts for less than 30 seconds and ends spontaneously.

Ventricular tachycardia is considered repetitive or recurrent if three or more discrete episodes are documented, while chronic ventricular tachycardia is that in which recurrent episodes occur for over a month.

As three or more ventricular premature complexes (VPCs) constitute ventricular tachycardia (VT), the causes of VT are similar to those of VPCs.

Causes of non-sustained ventricular tachycardia are:

- Pharmacological agents
  - Theophylline
  - Sympathomimetics
- Acute myocardial insult
  - Ischemia
  - Reperfusion
- Metabolic disorder
  - Hypoxia
  - Acidosis
  - Hypokalemia
- Cardiac trauma
  - Surgical
  - Accidental
  - Catheterization
- Drug intoxication
  - Digitalis
  - Quinidine

Sustained ventricular tachycardia is more often based on structural heart disease where a fixed anatomical substrate facilitates a re-entrant mechanism.

Causes of sustained ventricular tachycardia are:

- Myocardial scar
  - Infarction
  - Aneurysm

- Myocardial disease
  - Cardiomyopathy
  - Myocarditis
- Congestive failure
  - Ischemic
  - Hypertensive
- Valvular abnormality
  - Rheumatic heart disease
  - Mitral valve prolapse

Symptoms due to ventricular tachycardia depend on:

- The ventricular rate
- The duration of tachycardia
- Presence or absence of heart disease
- Severity of heart disease if it is present

Symptoms of sustained ventricular tachycardia with underlying heart disease and their causation are:

- Palpitation (fast heart rate)
- Angina (increased oxygen demand and shortened coronary filling time).
- Dyspnoea (pulmonary oedema due to loss of atrial contribution to ventricular filling)
- Syncope (low cardiac output state).

Clinical signs often observed during sustained ventricular tachycardia are:

- *Pulse* Fast and irregular pulse
- *BP* Low systolic blood pressure
- *JVP* Raised jugular venous pressure
- *Heart sounds* Systolic murmur and S_3 gallop.

The prognosis of sustained ventricular tachycardia depends upon the seriousness of the underlying cardiac disease particularly severity of coronary disease and degree of left ventricular dysfunction. The prognosis is particularly poor in ventricular tachycardia developing after acute myocardial infarction.

Markers of electrical instability in survivors of acute myocardial infarction are:

- Documented serious ventricular arrhythmias on 24 hour ambulatory Holter monitoring
- Reproducible sustained ventricular tachycardia on programmed electrical stimulation
- Late depolarization potentials detected on signal averaged electrocardiogram

The management of ventricular tachycardia depends upon the following factors:

- Sustained/non-sustained tachycardia
- Symptomatic/asymptomatic tachycardia
- Presence/absence of heart disease
- Presence/absence of cardiac decompensation.

The modalities of treatment of ventricular tachycardia are pharmacological, electrical and surgical.

- **Pharmacological therapy** Non-sustained ventricular tachycardia in an asymptomatic individual without organic heart disease only requires withdrawal of sympathomimetic drugs, and correction of any metabolic disorder or electrolyte imbalance.

  If the ventricular tachycardia is sustained and symptomatic, sympathetic stimulation by stress, exercise or adrenergic drugs is the most common cause, in the absence of heart disease. Such patients respond well to diltiazem and metoprolol.

If sustained symptomatic ventricular tachycardia occurs in the presence of organic heart disease, the line of treatment depends upon the haemodynamic status. All such patients are best managed in an intensive cardiac care unit under the expert guidance of a cardiologist.

If the haemodynamics are stable, pharmacological anti-arrhythmic therapy is initiated. The drugs of choice are lidocaine and amiodarone. First, a bolus dose of the drug is administered intravenously to be followed by a maintenance infusion.

The protocol of IV drug therapy of VT is:
Amiodarone 150 mg IV over 10 min (15 mg/min): repeat 150 mg IV every 10 min as needed.

OR

Lidocaine 0.5-0.75 mg/kg IV; repeat 0.5-0.75 mg/kg IV every 5-10 min as needed to a maximum of 3 mg/kg.

Once sinus rhythm is restored, an infusion of the rhythm converting drug is initiated as:

Amiodarone 360 mg IV over next 6 hrs (1 mg/min); maintain at 540 mg IV over next 18 hrs (0.5 mg/min)

OR

Lidocaine 2-4 mg/min (30-60 μg/kg/min).

Once the crisis period has been tided over, oral maintenance treatment with amiodarone may be instituted to prevent recurrence. Alternative drugs are flecainide, phenytoin, propafenone and sotalol.

Although one of these drugs may be used empirically, the ideal method is to select one of these drugs after electrophysiological study.

The drug that renders the ventricular tachycardia non-inducible by programmed electrical stimulation, is the one most likely to prevent recurrence of ventricular tachycardia.

- **Electrical cardioversion** If the haemodynamics are compromised with hypotension, myocardial ischemia, congestive heart failure and cerebral hypoperfusion, the ventricular tachycardia needs prompt termination by cardioversion.

An electrical shock of 50 to 100 J is the procedure of choice. It may be repeated with increasing energy of shock till sinus rhythm is restored. If to begin with, there is circulatory collapse and the peripheral pulses are not palpable, the initial dose of the DC shock should be 200 to 360 J.

Once sinus rhythm has been restored, long-term oral pharmacological treatment may be initiated.

- **Electrical pacing** A polymorphic ventricular tachycardia associated with a prolonged QT interval responds well to overdrive ventricular pacing.

  This arrhythmia is sometimes also treated with magnesium infusion or isoproterenol infusion.

- **Surgical treatment** Since a fixed anatomic substrate such as myocardial scar from previous infarction is often the basis of recurrent ventricular tachycardia, a surgical procedure can be offered for permanent cure.

  Surgical techniques available are endocardial resection and encircling ventriculotomy.

CHAPTER 20

Normal Regular Rhythm with Wide QRS Complexes

NORMAL WIDE-QRS RHYTHM

A regular cardiac rhythm at a rate of 60 to 100 beats per minute is considered to be a normal rhythm.

If the QRS complexes during such a rhythm are wide, it indicates abnormal intraventricular conduction of the impulses from the S-A node. The P waves and the QRS complexes during sinus rhythm maintain a 1:1 relationship with each other.

The well-known causes of wide QRS complexes during sinus rhythm are bundle branch block, intraventricular conduction defect and WPW syndrome. There is one more condition where wide QRS complexes arise from a ventricular pacemaker at a rate of 60 to 100 beats/min and is known as accelerated idioventricular rhythm (AIVR).

Let us see how this rhythm differs from sinus rhythm with wide QRS complexes.

ACCELERATED IDIOVENTRICULAR RHYTHM

Accelerated idioventricular rhythm (AIVR) is an ectopic rhythm originating from a latent subsidiary pacemaker located in the ventricular myocardium. Normally, such a pacemaker is subdued when the cardiac rhythm is governed by the S-A node.

However, when a ventricular pacemaker undergoes enhancement of its inherent automaticity, it produces an idioventricular rhythm. Since the heart rate during such rhythm exceeds the inherent ventricular rate, it is known as accelerated idioventricular rhythm (AIVR).

AIVR produces a regular rhythm at a rate of 60 to 100 beats/min that is greater than the inherent rate of the ventricular pacemaker which is 20-40 beats/min. The QRS complexes are bizarre and wide because of ventricular origin of the rhythm (Fig. 20.1).

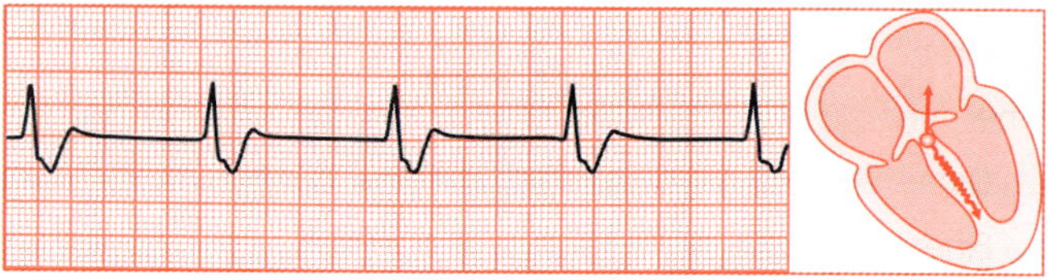

Fig. 20.1: Accelerated idioventricular rhythm (AIVR): slow wide QRS complexes

The distinctive feature of AIVR is atrioventricular dissociation or lack of relationship between the P waves and the QRS complexes. This is because, while the ventricles are activated by the ventricular pacemaker, the atria continue to be activated by the S-A node.

AIVR can be differentiated from ventricular tachycardia only by the ventricular rate. The rate is 60 to 100 beats/min in AIVR and 150 to 200 beats/min in VT, although both rhythms originate from the ventricles.

Clinical Relevance of a Regular Wide-QRS Rhythm

Sinus Rhythm with Wide QRS Complexes

A normal sinus rhythm, when associated with an intraventricular conduction defect, produces wide QRS complexes. The morphology of the QRS complex depends upon the cause of the conduction abnormality. Importantly, the 1:1 P-QRS relationship is maintained during sinus rhythm.

The significance of wide QRS complexes during sinus rhythm depends upon the cause of QRS widening. This has been discussed at length while dealing with abnormalities of the QRS complex.

Accelerated Idioventricular Rhythm

AIVR is most often observed in coronary care units in a setting of acute myocardial infarction. It either occurs spontaneously or as a reperfusion arrhythmia after thrombolytic therapy.

Other infrequent causes of AIVR are:

- Digitalis toxicity
- Rheumatic carditis
- Cardiac surgery

The above causes of AIVR are quite akin to those of a junctional tachycardia or accelerated idiojunctional rhythm. Both are examples of an idiofocal tachycardia.

AIVR is most often picked up from the monitor screen of an intensive coronary care unit (ICCU). It needs to be differentiated from its more serious counterpart ventricular tachycardia that often produces haemodynamic embarrassment, carries a poor prognosis and requires aggressive management. AIVR differs from VT, only in terms of the ventricular rate.

AIVR also needs to be differentiated from bundle branch block of recent onset, which is not uncommon in an ICCU setting. While AIVR produces bizarre and wide QRS complexes unrelated to P waves, bundle branch block is associated with a triphasic QRS contour and a maintained P-QRS relationship.

AIVR is usually asymptomatic as it occurs at the same rate-range as sinus rhythm. It rarely causes serious haemodynamic embarrassment. Only the loss of atrial contribution to ventricular filling (A-V dissociation) causes slight fall in cardiac output.

AIVR is usually transient and does not herald the onset of serious ventricular arrhythmias. Therefore, it is considered to be a benign arrhythmia with an excellent prognosis.

Active treatment of AIVR is generally not required as it is transient, asymptomatic and has few haemodynamic consequences. The hallmark of management of AIVR is constant observation. If treatment is required, it is only in patients with poor left ventricular function.

Atropine can be administered to accelerate the sinus rate, overdrive the ventricular rhythm and eliminate atrioventricular dissociation. Antiarrhythmic drugs, DC cardioversion and artificial pacing are unnecessary in the management of accelerated idioventricular rhythm.

CHAPTER 21

Fast Irregular Rhythm with Bizarre QRS Complexes

IRREGULAR WIDE-QRS RHYTHM

A cardiac rhythm that exceeds a rate of 100 beats per minute indicates a rapid discharge of impulses from the pacemaker governing the rhythm of the heart.

If the QRS complexes during such a rhythm are wide, bizarre looking and occur irregularly, it indicates a grossly abnormal pattern of intraventricular conduction and that the pacemaker is located in the ventricular myocardium.

Let us examine the specific arrhythmias that are associated with these features.

VENTRICULAR FLUTTER

Ventricular flutter is a fast ventricular rhythm produced either due to rapid discharge of impulses from a ventricular pacemaker or repetitive circus movement of an impulse in a re-entrant circuit. Therefore, ventricular flutter is quite akin to ventricular tachycardia in terms of its mechanism.

The heart rate in ventricular flutter is 150 to 200 beats per minute and is irregular. The QRS complexes are very wide and bizarre in morphology while the P waves and T waves are not visible (Fig. 21.1).

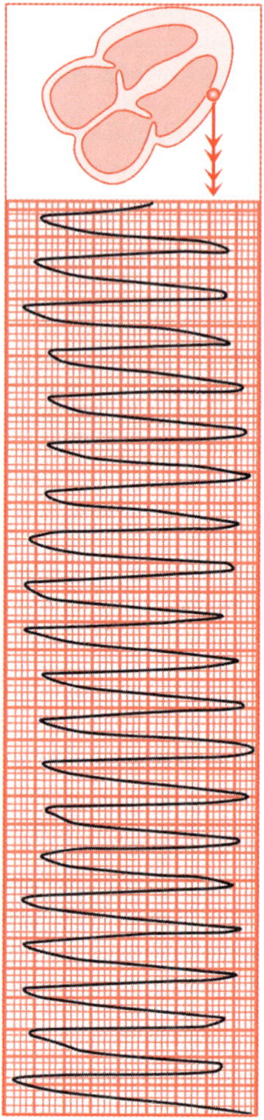

Fig. 21.1: Ventricular flutter: undulating large waves, no QRS-T distinction

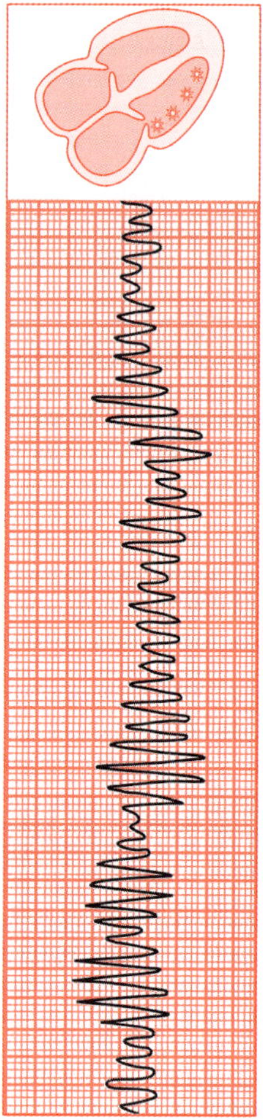

Fig. 21.2: Ventricular fibrillation: irregular, bizarre and chaotic deflections

In fact, merging of QRS complexes and T deflections produces a sine wave form. This is the differentiating feature from ventricular tachycardia where QRS complexes and T waves are identifiable separately.

The deflections in ventricular flutter although wide and bizarre, are large, constant in morphology and occur with slight irregularity. On the other hand, the deflections in ventricular fibrillation are relatively small, grossly variable in shape, height and width occurring in a totally chaotic fashion.

VENTRICULAR FIBRILLATION

Ventricular fibrillation is a grossly irregular rapid ventricular rhythm produced by a series of incoordinated and chaotic ventricular depolarizations.

Instead of the ventricles being activated systematically through the conduction system to produce coordinated pumping, the ventricular myocardium is functionally fractionated into numerous tissue islets in various stages of excitation and recovery. Ventricular depolarization is thus chaotic and ineffectual in producing haemodynamic pumping.

Ventricular fibrillation manifests with rapidly and irregularly occurring small deformed deflections that are grossly variable in shape, height and width. The regular waveforms of P waves, QRS complexes and T waves cannot be identified and the isoelectric line seems to waver unevenly (Fig. 21.2).

Ventricular fibrillation can be differentiated from ventricular flutter by the fact that in the latter condition, although the QRS complexes are bizarre and wide, they are relatively large, constant in morphology and occur only with slight irregularity.

Ventricular fibrillation needs to be differentiated from complete cardiac arrest or asystole in which no ECG deflections are recorded. This is possible by the fact that no matter how small, some definite deflections are always recorded in ventricular fibrillation.

Clinical Relevance of a Fast Irregular Bizarre-QRS Rhythm

Ventricular Flutter

Ventricular flutter is very similar to ventricular tachycardia in terms of mechanism and causation. In fact, even their ECG features closely resemble each other and at times they are indistinguishable.

Nevertheless, conversion of ventricular tachycardia to ventricular flutter is often associated with a precipitous fall in cardiac output and blood pressure.

Most often, ventricular flutter is a very transient arrhythmia as it frequently and rapidly degenerates into ventricular fibrillation. Therefore, ventricular flutter is most often picked up during cardiac monitoring in intensive care units.

Since ventricular flutter almost always converts to ventricular fibrillation, it is the treatment of the latter condition that is required.

Ventricular Fibrillation

Ventricular fibrillation is the most feared of all arrhythmias. It is often a terminal catastrophic event with an exceedingly poor prognosis and invariable progression to death if untreated. It is also the most common cause of sudden cardiac death.

Primary ventricular fibrillation occurs in a patient who does not have pre-existing hypotension or heart failure while secondary ventricular fibrillation occurs in those who have these abnormalities. Underlying advanced myocardial disease is invariable in those who develop secondary ventricular fibrillation.

Local cellular and metabolic factors that predispose to ventricular fibrillation are hypoxia, acidosis, hypoglycemia, hyperkalemia, catecholamine excess and accumulation of free fatty acids or lactates.

Frequent causes of ventricular fibrillation are:

- Myocardial infarction
    - Acute
    - Old

- Severe cardiomyopathy
  - Idiopathic
  - Ischemic
- Drug intoxication
  - Digitalis
  - Quinidine
- Metabolic derangement
  - Hypoxia
  - Acidosis
- Accidental event
  - Electrical shock
  - Hypothermia

Arrhythmias that are potentially serious as they may degenerate into ventricular fibrillation are:

- Ventricular tachycardia at more than 180 beats/min
- Ventricular tachycardia with supervening ischemia
- Torsade de pointes due to prolonged Q-T interval
- VPCs demonstrating 'R on T' phenomenon
- Atrial fibrillation with an accessory pathway.

Differentiation between ventricular flutter and ventricular fibrillation is generally a futile exercise as flutter is transient and almost always degenerates into ventricular fibrillation.

Clinically, it may be difficult to differentiate between ventricular fibrillation and cardiac standstill or asystole as both conditions cause absence of peripheral pulses and heart sounds with loss of consciousness.

Nevertheless, their distinction is crucial since defibrillation is required for ventricular fibrillation while external pacing is the mainstay of treatment for cardiac asystole.

The prognosis of ventricular fibrillation is exceedingly poor with invariable progress to death unless promptly treated. Prompt recognition and institution of defibrillation within a minute is the cornerstone of successful resuscitation.

Therefore, the prognosis of ventricular fibrillation is better in intensive care units and operation theatres with cardiac monitoring facility than elsewhere.

Many victims of acute myocardial infarction can be salvaged by training paramedical personnel and even laymen in the technique of cardiopulmonary resuscitation.

Moreover, mortality from myocardial infarction has declined in recent years through availability of intensive coronary care units (ICCUs) including mobile CCUs. These units are equipped with facilities for prompt recognition and cardioversion of serious ventricular arrhythmias such as ventricular fibrillation.

The moment ventricular fibrillation is recognized, the immediate goal should be to restore an effective cardiac rhythm. If defibrillation equipment is not available, a vigorous blow may be given to the precordium. This is popularly known as 'thump version' and may occasionally succeed in restoring sinus rhythm.

If not, cardiopulmonary resuscitation (CPR) should be begun immediately and the patient should be shifted to a hospital with defibrillation facility, in the minimum possible time.

The likelihood of success of defibrillation declines rapidly with time and irreversible brain damage occurs within four minutes of circulatory collapse.

Electrical defibrillation with 200 to 360 Joules of DC shock is the procedure of choice for the treatment of ventricular fibrillation. Longer the duration of fibrillation, higher is the energy level of shock required.

If one attempt fails, defibrillation may be repeated after intravenous bicarbonate 1 mEq/kg to correct the underlying acidosis, which increases the success rate of cardioversion.

If repeated attempts at defibrillation fail, intravenous drugs should be given 30-60 sec after each attempt. The dose of antiarrhythmic drugs that can be given is amiodarone 300 mg or lidocaine 1.0-1.5 mg/kg.

Recurrence of ventricular fibrillation can be prevented by anti-arrhythmic drugs used for prevention of ventricular tachycardia. Drugs that are used include flecainide, phenytoin, propafenone and sotalol.

Implantable defibrillators are now available, which when given to an ambulatory patient, can automatically sense ventricular fibrillation and deliver an electrical shock. The device is known as Automatic Implantable Cardioverter Defibrillator or AICD.

CHAPTER 22 Slow Regular Rhythm with Narrow QRS Complexes

REGULAR SLOW RHYTHM

A regular cardiac rhythm that occurs at a rate of less than 60 beats per minute indicates two broad possibilities:

- Slow discharge of impulses from the pacemaker governing the rhythm of the heart
- Block of alternate beats so that the conducted beats appear to occur at a slow rate

If the discharge rate of impulses is slow, the focus of impulse origin may be:

- Sinoatrial (S-A) node
- Junctional pacemaker

If alternate beats are blocked, the block may be:

- Sinoatrial (S-A) block
- Atrioventricular (A-V) block
- Blocked atrial ectopic beats

Narrow QRS complexes during such a rhythm indicate normal intraventricular conduction of impulses from a supraventricular pacemaker.

Let us examine the specific arrhythmias that are associated with these features.

SINUS BRADYCARDIA

The occurrence of sinus node discharge at a rate of less than 60 beats/min constitutes sinus bradycardia (Fig. 22.1).

In other words, the R-R interval exceeds 25 mm (heart rate = 1500/>25 = < 60). The rhythm is regular and the P wave and QRS morphology as well as P-QRS relationship are obviously as in normal sinus rhythm.

JUNCTIONAL ESCAPE RHYTHM

Junctional rhythm originates from a latent subsidiary pacemaker located in the A-V junction. Normally, this pacemaker is subdued, when the cardiac rhythm is governed by the S-A node. However, if the S-A node is at fault (sinus pause or sinus arrest), this junctional pacemaker takes charge of the cardiac rhythm.

Junctional rhythm is an example of escape rhythm since the junctional pacemaker escapes the subduing influence of the S-A node on the expression of its automaticity.

A junctional rhythm occurs at a rate of 40 to 60 beats/min which is the inherent rate of the junctional pacemaker (Fig. 22.2).

The distinctive feature of a junctional rhythm is the typical relationship between P waves and QRS complexes. As the atria are activated retrogradely, the P waves are inverted. They may just precede, just follow or be buried in the QRS complexes because of nearly simultaneous atrial and ventricular activation.

These characteristics of a junctional rhythm help to differentiate it from sinus bradycardia where the P waves are upright and always precede the QRS complexes by a fixed P-R interval.

SINUS RHYTHM WITH 2:1 S-A BLOCK

In second-degree sinoatrial block (2° S-A block), there is intermittent dropping of beats, resulting in pauses. In a dropped

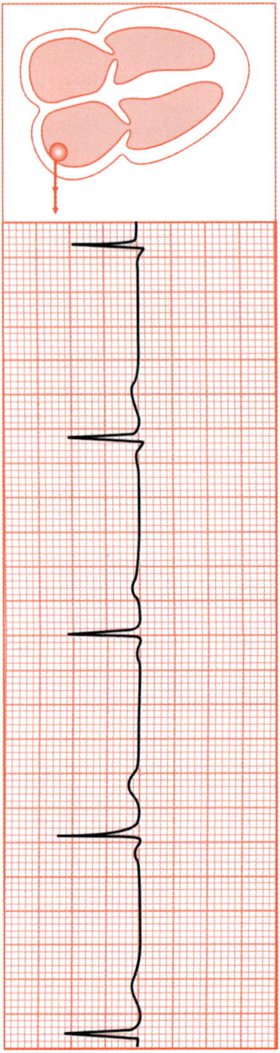

Fig. 22.1: Sinus bradycardia: heart rate less than 60/min (R-R > 25 mm)

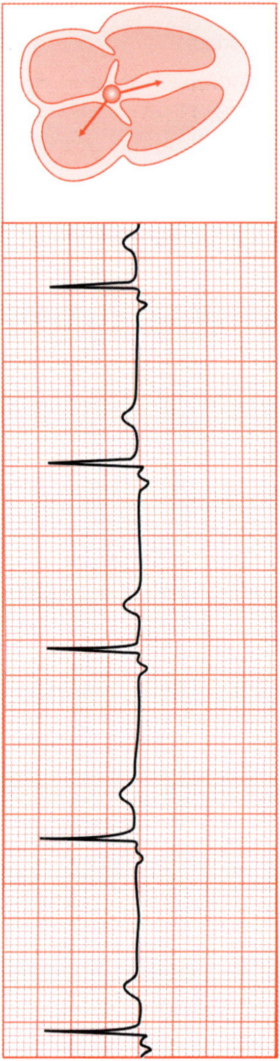

Fig. 22.2: Junctional rhythm: inverted P-wave precedes the QRS complex

beat, the entire P-QRS-T complex is missing as neither atrial nor ventricular activation occurs.

If the pattern of dropped beats is such that an alternate beat is missing (2:1 S-A block), the conducted beats resemble a slow regular rhythm such as sinus bradycardia.

The only difference is that if atropine is administered in 2:1 S-A block, there is a sudden doubling of the heart rate while in sinus bradycardia the heart rate accelerates gradually.

SINUS RHYTHM WITH 2:1 A-V BLOCK

In second-degree atrioventricular block (2° A-V block), there is intermittent dropping of ventricular complexes, resulting in pauses. In a dropped beat, the P-wave is not followed by a QRS complex as atrial activation is not followed by ventricular activation.

If the pattern of dropped beats is such that an alternate QRS complex is missing (2:1 A-V block), the normally conducted beats resemble a slow regular rhythm such as sinus bradycardia or 2:1 S-A block.

A 2:1 A-V block can be differentiated from 2:1 S-A block by the fact that P waves are recorded normally and only the QRS complexes are missing in alternate beats.

BLOCKED ATRIAL ECTOPICS IN BIGEMINY

An atrial premature complex (APC) inscribes a premature P-wave followed by a normal QRS complex and then a compensatory pause before the next sinus beat is recorded.

A very premature APC may find the A-V node still refractory to ventricular conduction and may consequently get blocked. Such an APC inscribes a P-wave that deforms the T-wave of the preceding beat, is not followed by a QRS complex but followed by a compensatory pause.

If such blocked APCs alternate with normal beats, the normal sinus beats resemble a slow regular rhythm such as sinus bradycardia or 2:1 S-A block.

The distinctive feature of blocked atrial ectopics in bigeminal rhythm is the occurrence of premature bizarre P-waves deforming the T-waves.

A 2:1 A-V block also produces blocked P-waves but they are not premature and are normal in morphology.

Clinical Relevance of a Slow Regular Narrow-QRS Rhythm

Sinus Bradycardia

Sinus bradycardia represents response of the S-A node to a variety of physiological and pathological stimuli mediated by the nervous and hormonal control over the rate of pacemaker discharge.

The causes of sinus bradycardia are:

- Advanced age and athletic built
- Deep sleep and hypothermia
- Raised intracranial tension or glaucoma
- Hypopituitarism or hypothyroidism
- Obstructive jaundice or uraemia
- Beta blockers and calcium blockers
- Sick sinus syndrome

Sinus bradycardia is usual in young vagotonic trained athletes and in elderly patients with a low sinus node discharge rate.

Sinus bradycardia during strenuous activity and in the absence of medical conditions or drugs likely to cause a slow heart rate is a sign of sinus-node dysfunction, the so called "sick sinus syndrome".

Sinus bradycardia is not a primary arrhythmia and therefore, treatment should be directed towards the basic underlying condition. Examples are hormone replacement in endocrinal disorders, decongestive therapy in high intracranial/intraocular tension, medical treatment of hepatic/renal disease and withdrawal of the offending drug in drug-induced sinus bradycardia.

Symptomatic sinus bradycardia in the absence of these conditions should be managed as sick sinus syndrome. Atropine and sympathomimetic drugs can temporarily accelerate the ventricular rate.

Junctional Rhythm

A junctional escape rhythm is a 'rescue' rhythm in which the junctional pacemaker is asked to govern the rhythm of the heart when the sinus node produces insufficient impulses due to severe bradycardia or S-A block.

The term 'escape' rhythm signifies that the junctional pacemaker has escaped the subduing influence of the dominant pacemaker, the S-A node. A junctional rhythm after sinus arrest is the body's defence mechanism against prolonged asystole.

Sinus Rhythm with 2:1 Block

A sinus rhythm in which alternate beats are blocked (2:1 block) closely resembles sinus bradycardia as the conducted beats appear to occur at a slow rate. The block may be either sinoatrial (S-A block) or atrioventricular (A-V block).

Sick sinus syndrome is a frequent cause of 2:1 S-A block next only to drugs that reduce the pacemaker discharge rate (e.g. propranolol, diltiazem).

The causes of 2:1 A-V block are acute carditis, drugs that cause 2:1 S-A block (see above) and inferior wall myocardial infarction.

In the management of symptomatic 2:1 block,drugs like atropine and adrenalin can temporarily accelerate the ventricular rate.

Temporary cardiac pacing is effective in tiding over the crisis in acute carditis, drug toxicity or myocardial infarction.

Permanent cardiac pacing is the answer to the management of sick sinus syndrome when symptoms are severe, recurrent and long-standing.

Blocked APCs in Bigeminal Rhythm

Atrial premature complexes that are blocked in the A-V node and alternate with sinus beats, resemble a slow rhythm. This occurs because of the compensatory pause that follows each premature beat.

Such a rhythm needs to be differentiated from other slow rhythms, the management of which is entirely different.

Blocked or non-conducted atrial premature beats are frequently observed in elderly patients who have advanced A-V nodal disease and in the presence of digitalis toxicity.

23 CHAPTER

Slow Irregular Rhythm with Narrow QRS Complexes

IRREGULAR SLOW RHYTHM

An irregular cardiac rhythm that occurs at a rate of less than 60 beats per minute indicates three possibilities:

- Slow and variable rate of pacemaker discharge.
- Beat-to-beat variability of the focus of origin.
- Varying degree of conduction block of regular beats.

Narrow QRS complexes during such a rhythm indicate normal intraventricular conduction of impulses from a supraventricular pacemaker.

Let us examine the specific arrhythmias that are associated with these features.

SINUS ARRHYTHMIA

Sinus arrhythmia is an irregular rhythm characterized by periods of slow and fast heart rate due to variation in the rate of SA node discharge.

When the periodic change in sinus rate is related to the phases of respiration, it is known as respiratory sinus arrhythmia. Non-respiratory sinus arrhythmia is where the sinus rate variability is uninfluenced by the respiratory cycle.

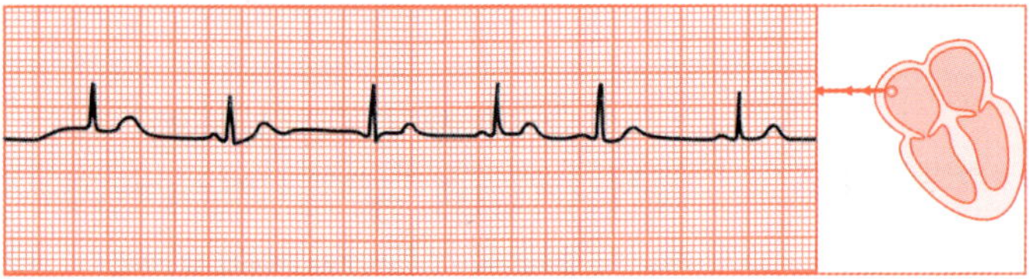

Fig. 23.1: Sinus arrhythmia: heart rate increases in inspiration and decreases in expiration

Sinus arrhythmia is characterized by alternating periods of long and short P-P and R-R intervals reflecting a variable heart rate (Fig. 23.1).

In respiratory sinus arrhythmia, about four complexes occur at one rate while the next four complexes occur at a different rate. The figure of 4 presumes that the respiratory rate is one-fourth of the heart rate. The rate is faster in inspiration and slower in expiration.

In non-respiratory sinus arrhythmia, the variability of heart rate is non-phasic and unrelated to respiration.

Since, all beats arise from the S-A node, the P-wave shape, QRS complex morphology and P-R interval are constant. Sinus arrhythmia is frequently associated with sinus bradycardia.

WANDERING PACEMAKER RHYTHM

Wandering pacemaker is a rhythm wherein, impulses take origin from different foci besides the S-A node. The pacemaker, so to say, wanders from one focus to the other, from beat-to-beat. The focus of origin may be the S-A node, the atrial myocardium or the A-V junction.

Wandering pacemaker rhythm is characterized by a beat-to-beat variability of the P-wave morphology (Fig. 23.2).

Upright P-waves arise from the SA node or upper atrium while inverted P waves arise from the lower atrium or A-V junction.

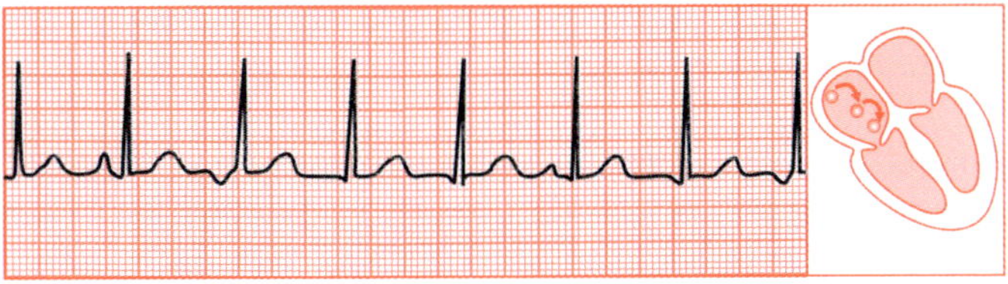

Fig. 23.2: Wandering pacemaker rhythm: varying P-wave morphology and changing P-R interval

The P-R interval also varies from beat-to-beat due to variability of the A-V conduction time. Lower atrial or junctional beats have a shorter P-R interval because of shorter conduction time.

This rhythm can be differentiated from sinus arrhythmia by the fact that the variability of heart rate is not phasic but on a beat-to-beat basis. Moreover, in sinus arrhythmia, the P-wave morphology and P-R interval are constant since all beats arise from the S-A node.

SINUS RHYTHM WITH VARYING S-A BLOCK

In second-degree sinoatrial block (2° S-A block), there is intermittent dropping of beats, resulting in pauses. In a dropped beat, the entire P-QRS-T complex is missing as neither atrial nor ventricular activation occurs.

The pattern of dropped beats determines the conduction ratio such as 2:1 S-A block if alternate beats are dropped, 3:2 if every third beat is dropped and so on. If the conduction ratio is variable, it produces a slow irregular rhythm.

SINUS RHYTHM WITH VARYING A-V BLOCK

In second-degree atrioventricular block (2° A-V block), there is intermittent dropping of ventricular complexes, resulting in pauses. In a dropped beat, the P-wave is not followed by a QRS complex as atrial activation is not followed by ventricular activation.

The ratio of the number of P waves to number of QRS complexes determines the conduction sequence such as 2:1 A-V block if alternate P-wave is blocked, 3:2 if every third P-wave is blocked and so on. If the conduction ratio is variable, it produces a slow irregular rhythm.

Varying A-V block can be differentiated from varying S-A block by the fact that P waves are recorded normally in A-V block. They are altogether missing along with the QRS complexes, in case of S-A block.

Clinical Relevance of a Slow Irregular Narrow–QRS Rhythm

Sinus Arrhythmia

Respiratory sinus arrhythmia is produced by variation in the vagal tone in relation to the respiratory cycle, caused by reflex mechanisms in the pulmonary and systemic vasculature. It is a normal physiological phenomenon often observed in children and young vagotonic individuals.

Non-respiratory sinus arrhythmia is an irregularity of heart rate produced by a dysfunctional S-A node in elderly patients, the so called sick sinus syndrome.

Since sinus arrhythmia results from variation in the vagal influence on the S-A node, it is accentuated by vagotonic procedures like carotid sinus pressure and abolished by vagolytic procedures such as exercise and atropine administration.

Absence of sinus arrhythmia with a clock-like regularity of the heart rate indicates absence of vagal influence on the S-A node and is a feature of autonomic neuropathy.

Respiratory sinus arrhythmia in children and young adults merits no active treatment. Non-respiratory sinus arrhythmia in the elderly is managed as sick sinus syndrome.

Wandering Pacemaker Rhythm

A cardiac rhythm due to a wandering pacemaker is a striking but benign electrocardiographic abnormality. It is often observed in young, asymptomatic and healthy individuals.

Occasionally, wandering pacemaker rhythm is observed during the course of digitalis treatment or acute rheumatic fever.

No active treatment is indicated in young asymptomatic persons in whom a wandering pacemaker rhythm is observed incidentally.

Management of digitalis toxicity or rheumatic carditis is indicated if these causes are implicated. Symptomatic bradycardia due to this rhythm is managed with atropine or sympathomimetics.

Sinus Rhythm with Varying Block

A sinus rhythm, when complicated by sinoatrial or atrioventricular block of a variable degree, produces an irregular heart rate.

Sick sinus syndrome is a frequent cause of varying S-A block. Variable A-V block is often due to rheumatic carditis or acute inferior wall infarction.

Slow Atrial Fibrillation

Atrial fibrillation generally produces a fast irregular ventricular rhythm. This is because, out of the large number of fibrillatory waves, only a few can randomly penetrate the A-V node and activate the ventricles producing a ventricular rate of 100 to 150 beats per minute.

In other words, atrial fibrillation is associated with a variable degree of physiological A-V block. If this physiological A-V block is advanced, the ventricular rate is slow, resulting in slow atrial fibrillation.

Slow atrial fibrillation is observed, if there is pre-existing A-V nodal disease or during treatment with drugs like propranolol, verapamil or diltiazem that block the AV node.

Atropine and sympathomimetic agents can temporarily accelerate the ventricular rate in symptomatic S-A or A-V block.

Temporary pacing is useful in the acute phase of carditis, drug intoxication or myocardial infarction. Permanent cardiac pacing is the answer to recurrent and severe symptoms due to sick sinus syndrome.

CHAPTER 24

Slow Regular Rhythm with Wide QRS Complexes

SLOW WIDE-QRS RHYTHM

A regular cardiac rhythm that occurs at a rate of less than 60 beats per minute indicates slow discharge of impulses from the pacemaker governing the rhythm of the heart.

If the QRS complexes during such a rhythm are wide, two possibilities have to be considered:

- The rhythm is ventricular in origin in which case ventricular activation is through myocardium and not the specialized conduction system.
- The rhythm is supraventricular in origin but there is a pre-existing abnormality causing wide QRS complexes.

A slow ventricular rhythm occurs in these situations:

- Complete A-V block with an idioventricular rhythm
- Complete S-A block with ventricular escape rhythm
- Ventricular rhythm from an implanted pacemaker.

Let us go into the classical features of these rhythms.

COMPLETE A-V BLOCK

In complete or third-degree atrioventricular block (3° A-V block), there is a total interruption of A-V conduction with the result that no sinus beat is able to activate the ventricles.

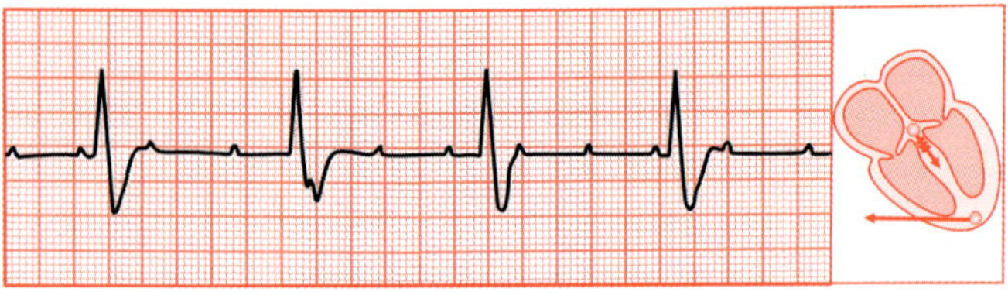

Fig. 24.1: Third-degree (complete) AV block: wide QRS complexes

Therefore, the ventricles are governed by a subsidiary pacemaker in the ventricular myocardium. The inherent rate of this pacemaker is 20 to 40 beats per minute and hence, the wide QRS complexes occur at this rate (Fig. 24.1).

However, since the atria continue to be activated by the S-A node, the P waves occur at a rate of 70 to 80 beats per minute. Since, the S-A node and the ventricular pacemaker are asynchronous and produce independent rhythms, there is no relationship between the P waves and QRS complexes. This is known as A-V dissociation.

The ventricular rhythm at its inherent rate of 20 to 40 beats per minute is called idioventricular rhythm.

Occasionally in complete A-V block, the ventricles are governed by a subsidiary pacemaker in the His bundle. The inherent rate of this pacemaker is 40 to 60 beats per minute and hence, the QRS complexes occur at this rate.

Moreover, since ventricular conduction proceeds through normal pathways, the QRS complexes may be narrow (Fig. 24.2).

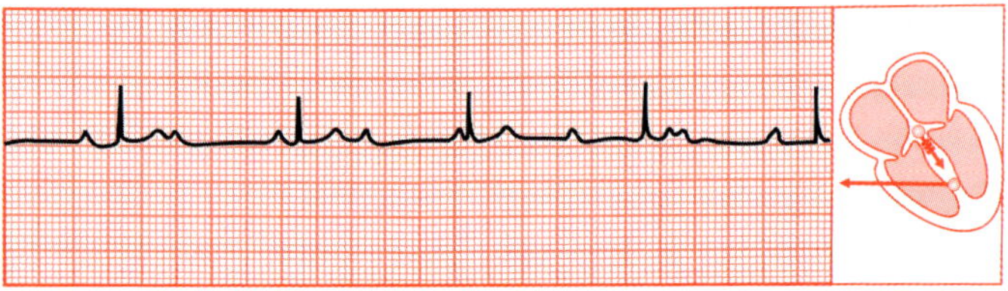

Fig. 24.2: Third-degree (complete) AV block: narrow QRS complexes

A His bundle rhythm closely resembles a junctional rhythm as both occur at the same rate and produce narrow QRS complexes.

The differentiating feature is that in His bundle rhythm of complete A-V block, the QRS complexes are unrelated to the P waves. In a junctional rhythm, the P waves just precede, just follow or are merged with the QRS complexes.

COMPLETE S-A BLOCK

In complete or third-degree sinoatrial block (3° S-A block), there is sinus node arrest or total atrial standstill with the result that ventricular activation is not possible.

Therefore, a subsidiary pacemaker comes to rescue by taking over the rhythm of the heart. Generally, it is the junctional pacemaker which governs the cardiac rhythm in this situation, producing a junctional escape rhythm.

However, if the A-V node is diseased, a ventricular pacemaker is called upon to govern the heart, producing a ventricular rhythm. The inherent rate of this pacemaker is 20 to 40 beats per minute and wide QRS complexes occur at this rate.

Since the ventricular pacemaker escapes the subduing influence of the S-A node on the expression of its automaticity, the rhythm is known as ventricular escape rhythm.

A ventricular escape rhythm in complete S-A block resembles the idioventricular rhythm in complete A-V block as both occur at a similar rate and produce wide QRS complexes.

They can be differentiated by the fact that normal P-waves at a rate of 70 to 80 beats continue to occur in A-V block. No signs of atrial activation are observed in S-A block and therefore P-waves are altogether absent.

ARTIFICIAL PACEMAKER RHYTHM

In complete S-A block or A-V block with a very slow heart rate, the definitive form of treatment is implanting an external pacemaker. Artificial pacing is generally done from the right ventricle. The pacemaker is programmed to deliver impulses at a predetermined rate of around 60 beats per minute.

These impulses are generated either continuously (fixed mode pacing) or intermittently (demand mode pacing) that is, only when the pacemaker senses an insufficient number of intrinsic impulses.

In either case, the pacemaker beats produce wide QRS complexes as the ventricles are activated asynchronously, right ventricular activation preceding the left. The heart rate depends upon the rate to which the pacemaker has been programmed.

The rhythm from an artificial pacemaker resembles an idioventricular rhythm of complete A-V block. The differentiating feature is a spike-like deflection before each QRS complex, known as pacemaker artefact (Fig. 24.3).

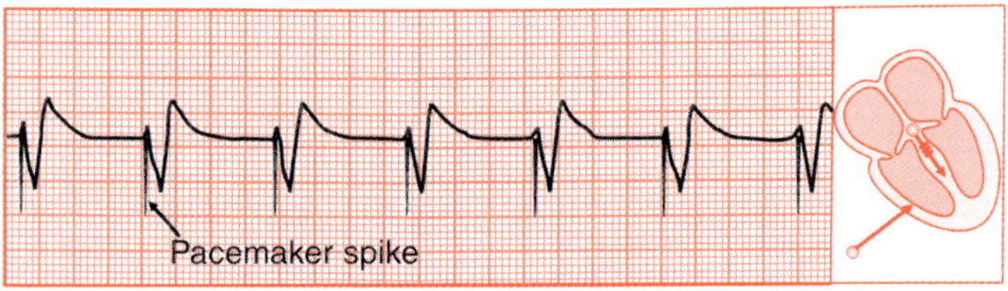

Fig. 24.3: Artificial pacemaker rhythm: spike before each QRS complex

SLOW RHYTHM WITH PRE-EXISTING QRS ABNORMALITY

It is known that certain conditions produce an abnormality of ventricular conduction even in sinus rhythm causing an alteration of QRS morphology.

Three well known examples are:

- Bundle branch block
- WPW syndrome
- Intraventricular conduction defect

If a slow supraventricular rhythm such as sinus bradycardia occurs in the presence of a pre-existing QRS abnormality, it is naturally associated with wide QRS complexes.

A bundle branch block produces a triphasic QRS contour while an intraventricular conduction defect results in a bizarre QRS morphology. The WPW syndrome is characterized by a delta wave on the ascending limb of the QRS complex.

Clinical Relevance of a Slow Regular Wide-QRS Rhythm

Complete A-V Block

The causes of complete or third-degree AV block are:

- Congenital heart disease, e.g. septal defect
- Coronary disease, e.g. inferior wall infarction
- Cardiac surgery, e.g. atrial septal repair
- Aortic valve disease, e.g. calcific stenosis
- Fibrocalcerous degeneration, e.g. Lev's disease.

In complete A-V block, the ventricles are governed by a subsidiary pacemaker in the His bundle or the ventricular myocardium. While a His bundle rhythm produces narrow QRS complexes at 40 to 60 beats/min, a ventricular rhythm produces wide QRS complexes at 20 to 40 beats/min.

A His bundle rhythm is more stable, reliable to sustain ventricular function, can be accelerated by atropine and rarely causes symptoms. On the other hand, a ventricular rhythm is unstable, unreliable to sustain ventricular function, cannot be accelerated by atropine and often causes syncope.

Clinical importance of A-V block depends upon:

- Causes of the A-V block: reversible or irreversible
- Site of the lower pacemaker: His bundle or ventricle
- Symptomatology of the patient: present or absent

The most common symptom of complete A-V block is spells of dizziness or fainting due to transient ventricular asystole with sudden decline in cardiac output. Such episodes or syncopal attacks are known as Stokes-Adam's attacks.

Other causes of Stokes-Adam's attacks are:

- Complete sinoatrial block
- Serious ventricular arrhythmia
- Carotid sinus hypersensitivity
- Subclavian steal syndrome

It is extremely important to differentiate Stokes-Adam's attack due to complete A-V block from that due to a ventricular arrhythmia as their management is entirely different. While asystole requires atropine or cardiac pacing, ventricular arrhythmia requires antiarrhythmic drugs or electrical cardioversion.

Complete A-V block produces the following clinical signs that help to differentiate it from other slow rhythms:

- Dissociation of jugular venous waves from carotid arterial pulsations, due to A-V dissociation
- Variable intensity of the first heart sound, due to variable duration of diastolic filling period.

Cardiac pacing is the definitive form of treatment in complete A-V block. While temporary pacing may be enough to tide over a transient situation such as an acute myocardial infarction or a postoperative complication, permanent pacing is the answer to a chronic condition like calcific degeneration of the A-V node.

Pacing is invariably required in these situations:

- Wide QRS rhythm at less than 40 beats/min
- History of recurrent Stokes-Adam's attacks
- Setting of an acute myocardial infarction.

Complete S-A Block

The causes of complete or third-degree SA block are:

- Drug therapy, e.g. propranolol, digitalis, diltiazem
- Vagal stimulation, e.g. by carotid sinus pressure
- Sinus node dysfunction, e.g. sick sinus syndrome.

In complete S-A block, the ventricles are governed by a subsidiary pacemaker in the A-V junction or the ventricular myocardium. While a junctional rhythm produces narrow QRS complexes at 40 to 60 beats/min, a ventricular rhythm produces wide QRS complexes at 20 to 40 beats/min.

Both these rhythms are examples of an escape rhythm, since the subsidiary pacemaker escapes the subduing influence of the S-A node on the expression of its automaticity. A ventricular escape rhythm occurs only if the A-V node is diseased and cannot govern the cardiac rhythm.

Sinoatrial block may co-exist with atrioventricular block and even right or left bundle branch block especially in elderly individuals with a diffuse fibrocalcerous or degenerative process involving the entire conduction system.

The escape rhythm in complete S-A block is a "rescue" rhythm in the absence of which prolonged asystole would invariably result in death.

The most common symptom of complete S-A block is spells of dizziness or fainting due to transient ventricular asystole along with sudden decline in cardiac output. S-A block in one of the causes of Stokes-Adam's attacks.

Treatment of symptomatic individuals involves administration of drugs like atropine and sympathomimetic drugs to accelerate the heart rate. The dosages of these drugs used are:

Atropine 0.6 mg IV; repeat every 3-5 min upto response or a total dose of 0.03-0.04 mg/kg

OR

Epinephrine 1 mg IV (10 ml of 1:10000 solution)

Cardiac pacing remains the definitive form of treatment of complete S-A block. When the S-A block is a part of sick sinus syndrome, the management of that condition is indicated.

Artificial Pacemaker Rhythm

The artificial pacemaker is an electronic device that can generate impulses to activate the heart, if the intrinsic rhythm is slow or unstable. Generally, the pacemaker lead with the electrode at its tip is implanted on the endocardial surface of the right ventricle.

External pacing may be employed temporarily to tide over an acute transient situation or permanently in a chronic condition.

There are two modes of cardiac pacing namely, fixed–mode pacing and demand-mode pacing.

In fixed-mode pacing, impulses are generated at a predetermined rate, irrespective of the intrinsic rhythm. In demand-mode pacing, the pacemaker generates impulses intermittently on demand, when it senses a slow intrinsic rhythm.

When an external pacemaker governs the cardiac rhythm, the ventricles are not activated synchronously but sequentially. The right ventricle is activated before the left since the pacing electrode is located in the right ventricle.

Therefore, an artificial pacemaker rhythm is characterized by wide QRS complexes. The rate of the pacemaker rhythm is the rate at which the pacemaker has been programmed.

Slow Rhythm with Pre-existing QRS Abnormality

The occurrence of a slow rhythm in a patient who has a pre-existing condition causing wide QRS complexes such as bundle branch block or conduction defect, understandably simulates an idioventricular rhythm.

The availability of a previous ECG during normal sinus rhythm that reveals wide QRS complexes can settle the issue.

Moreover, the triphasic contour of a bundle branch block or the delta wave of WPW syndrome are too characteristic to be mistaken for the wide QRS complexes of a ventricular rhythm.

INDEX

A

B

C

D

E

F

H

I

J

L

M

N

P

Q

R

S

T

V

W